MASSAC

MASSAGE

KEN EYERMAN

PHOTOGRAPHS BY

ANTHONY CRICKMAY AND ROB HAINES

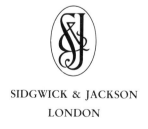

SIDGWICK & JACKSON

LONDON

First published in Great Britain in 1987 by
Sidgwick & Jackson Limited
1 Tavistock Chambers, Bloomsbury Way
London WC1A 2SG

ISBN 0 283 99406 1

Phototypeset by Falcon Graphic Art Limited
Wallington, Surrey
Printed in Great Britain by
Butler & Tanner Limited

Note Always observe the cautions in this book and, if you are
in doubt about any of the exercises because of a medical
condition, do not attempt them.

CONTENTS

ACKNOWLEDGEMENTS

I'd like to thank the following for their invaluable help on this book: Chris Bannerman, Veronica Bodnarec, Paul Bowden, Chiggy, Anthony Crickmay, Steven Daniels, Annabel Edwards, Victoria Eldon, Rob Haines, Celia Hulton, Tony Mellor, Terry Ross, Lizie Saunderson and Philip Simon.

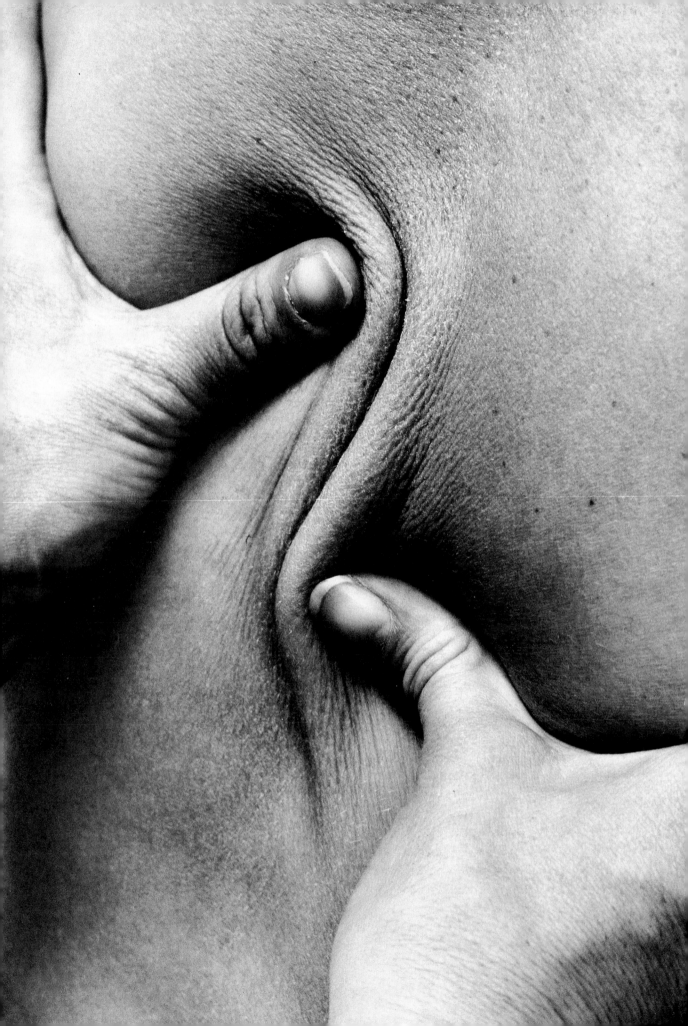

INTRODUCTION

Massage is often dismissed as having only superficial value: a general treatment to relax tight muscles and to give temporary relief from emotional tension. It can, however, be of a more fundamental benefit, both to the giver and the receiver.

Massage is a way to rediscover the body through touch. This physical contact is important for learning and change – it often takes someone else's energy and touch to bring problems to the surface. The first step in freeing emotional or muscular tension is to make ourselves more aware of its existence.

These ideas are vital to an understanding of the massage technique I describe in this book. My own interest in massage stems from two experiences which taught me how little I really knew about my own body and which introduced me to the two massage techniques, one Western, one Eastern, that have influenced my own approach.

About fifteen years ago, whilst I was studying contemporary dance in California, I went on a visit to New York. A friend gave me a massage treatment, specially designed for the needs of dancers, based on the work of Alfred Kagan. Unlike the physically superficial massage techniques, such as Swedish massage, this worked deep in the body, lengthening and balancing the muscles, always working in line with their correct anatomical direction. As a dancer, I considered my body to be perfectly fit and co-ordinated, working to its full potential. But I was suddenly made aware of how tight and disconnected it really was. My muscles were unevenly developed, causing tension and a lack of balance – and up to this point I was so out of touch with my body I had not even noticed.

About the same time as this, I attended a class concerned with the creation and role of energy in the body, based on the polarity therapy of the American osteopath, Dr Randolph Stone. It centred on Eastern principles and combined a vegetarian diet, herbal remedies, manipulation and gentle exercises. This soft, introspective approach was in complete contrast to the forceful, outward expression of my dance training. In fact, it changed my life. I became aware of feelings on a far more subtle level than I had known before. I needed fewer hours sleep and had much more energy.

These two experiences made me realize that massage was the way to work with the body at the most fundamental level. My interest in massage has thus grown into a way of life based on both Western and Eastern concepts.

BALANCE

The idea that links the two is that of balance. In the West the aim of massage is to achieve balance by working on the physical structure of the body.

The skeleton is supported by a multi-layered web of soft tissue: muscles, ligaments, tendons, etc. When we made the transition from four-legged to two-legged creatures, we freed the upper body for expression, leaving the lower body to generate power for propulsion. This left the body unstable, constantly having to struggle to stay upright, aligned and balanced against the downward pull of gravity. Western massage works on the soft tissue, strengthening and balancing it. It helps to ensure that the right muscles are doing the right work; that, for instance, the muscles of the abdominal wall are not being strained by being used to support the weight of the spine and the upper body because the deeper muscles surrounding the spine are too weak to fulfil this supportive function. Western massage works to lengthen the spine, giving upward lift and direction, and to keep the pelvis, legs and feet – what Dr Ida Rolf* calls the 'underpinning' – working correctly. The pelvis, which forms the connection between the energy-generating lower limbs and the expressive upper body, should be horizontally balanced and the feet and legs firm and supportive.

Thus the Western technique relates to the body's structure, alignment, habit and movement. The strokes work deeply and anatomically correctly, following the line of the muscles. It is designed to stimulate, relax, lengthen and balance the body structure by massaging the muscle groups in a systematic way. The technique re-educates the body, helping to locate the painful areas caused by poor movement habits. When the spine and its supporting structure are correctly aligned, breathing, circulation and digestion are all improved.

* Dr Ida Rolf initiated the now-famous Rolfing technique. By the process of physical manipulation, muscle tissue in the body is lengthened and the bones are allowed to readjust themselves to their proper place and their proper relation to each other. Ida Rolf started work in America but her technique is now used across the Western world.

The Eastern approach to massage is more inward-looking. The idea is to restore the free flow of energy around the body, connecting the inner body to the outer. Again the important aim is to achieve balance: the creation of harmony through the balance of the opposing energies, *yin* and *yang*.

The Chinese use the terms yin and yang to express their concept of the universe, of the way in which things relate to each other. They are complementary opposites, constantly changing in a dynamic interplay but always in relation to the whole. Yin represents the shady side of a slope and is associated with cold, dark, passive, inward and downward qualities. Yang is the sunny side of the slope. It is associated with hot, light, active, outward and upward qualities and movements. Thus the relationship between yin and yang is the relationship of dark to light, mother to father, feet to head, earth to spirit.

In massage we talk of an area of the body being dense, over-active or hot. This is a yang quality, whilst yin would be empty, under-active or cold. What we are trying to achieve is balance and harmony by softening and relaxing over-active areas, and bringing energy, warmth and activity to the weaker areas. Chinese medicine is based on this concept of balancing opposing energies, and approaches healing as an art as well as a science. Its history and development date back more than 2000 years and are fundamentally bound up with Chinese culture and philosophy. It is also closely linked with nature; receptiveness and intuition are used in conjunction with scientific and rational principles.

SHIATSU

The Eastern technique that has influenced me most is Shiatsu. This is a deep massage technique developed in Japan but based on the theories of traditional Chinese medicine, the basic aim being the creation of harmony through the balancing of opposing energies. Energy, known by the Chinese as *chi*, is the essence of everything. Chi is said to flow around the body along pathways called meridians. The centre of energy is known as the *hara*. This is believed to be situated in the abdomen. It is the beginning point for the cyclic flow of energy. Each of the 12 meridians is associated with a particular organ; for example, there are bladder, gall bladder, kidney and stomach meridians. (See the diagram on p.12.) Along these pathways lie more than 350 acupressure points, although only about a hundred are used. Stimulating a point somewhere along the meridian relating to a particular organ will affect that organ, even if the point is nowhere near. Different parts of the body are also associated with specific organs. Shiatsu massage seeks to restore any imbalance in the energy flow by manipulation of these parts and points.

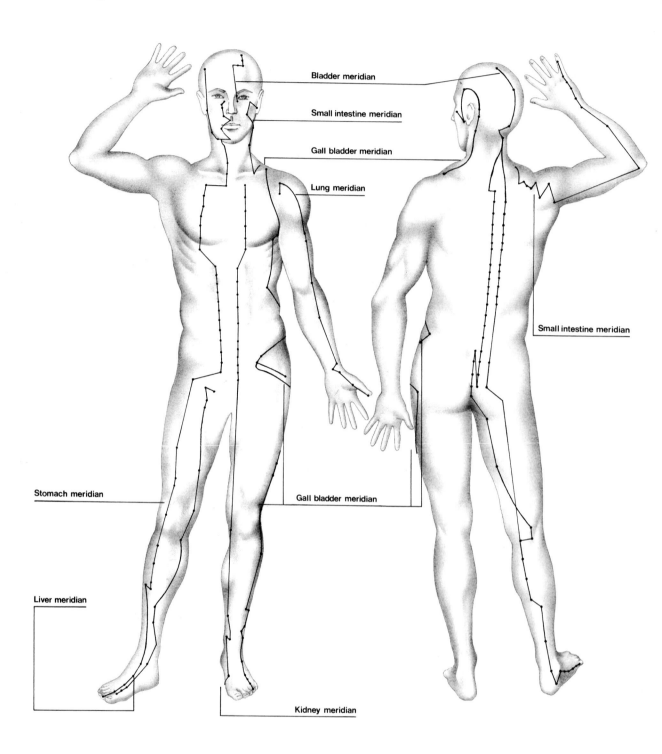

Bladder meridian

Small intestine meridian

Gall bladder meridian

Lung meridian

Small intestine meridian

Stomach meridian

Gall bladder meridian

Liver meridian

Kidney meridian

This illustration shows some of the 12 meridians used in Shiatsu. Each one is associated with a specific organ and stimulation of a point on the meridian will affect that organ

CONCLUSION

Thus from the East we learn to work on the body's inner core of energy to restore the efficiency of the organs and physical structure of the body as well as creating emotional and psychological balance. From the West we learn to benefit the mind and body by stimulating and balancing the outer tissue.

In this book, which is structured like a series of lessons, I describe how to combine these two approaches. The first chapter, Fundamental Energy, is the general introductory lesson in which I teach the principles of massage: how to begin breathing correctly and how to use weight and energy. The seven chapters following are all lessons on how to massage a certain area of the body. The order follows that of a general massage treatment: back, pelvis and back of legs, feet and front of legs, abdomen and chest, shoulders and arms and, finally, neck and face.

We usually start with the back in this way not only because it is the most important area, bearing more strain and stress than anywhere else, but also because it is the least personal part of the body to touch. As you work round the body in a logical sequence you will build up trust with your partner – that is, the person you are massaging – before beginning to massage the more sensitive abdomen and face.

At the end of some of the chapters there are exercises designed to make you relax and deepen your breathing as well as to improve the alignment and efficiency of your body. You and your partner may find it helpful to do a couple of these at the beginning of every session.

The final chapter is entitled Body Reading. As we become familiar with the human body from massaging it, we also become more aware, not only of our own bodies, but of those around us. Careful observation tells us a great deal about other people and also about ourselves. Body reading is not concerned with judging but with continuing this process of learning.

The book is designed to be visual and experiential. The photographs stand on their own as beautifully clear illustrations, expressing the essence of massage: its interplay of movement and stillness; its use of breath and focus; and its sensitivity and physicality, by which I mean the awareness of every part of your body, the sense of living in your whole body and not just your head.

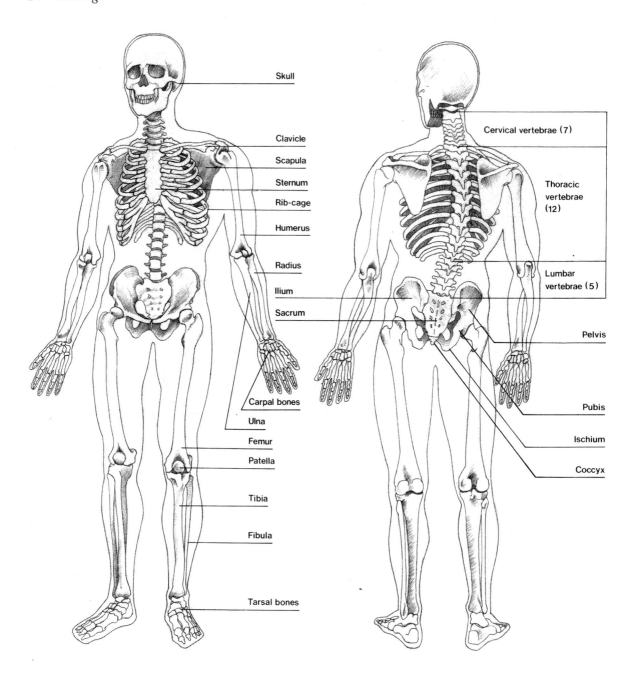

Skull

Clavicle

Scapula

Sternum

Rib-cage

Humerus

Radius

Ilium

Sacrum

Carpal bones

Ulna

Femur

Patella

Tibia

Fibula

Tarsal bones

Cervical vertebrae (7)

Thoracic vertebrae (12)

Lumbar vertebrae (5)

Pelvis

Pubis

Ischium

Coccyx

The bones form the basic structure of the body; they are linked by muscles and ligaments around the joints. The correct alignment of the body's structural system, in particular the spine, is essential for good health

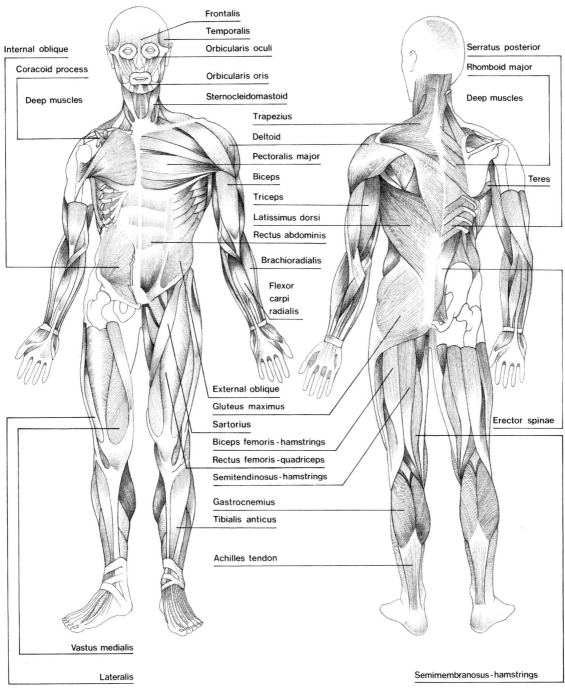

Frontalis
Temporalis
Orbicularis oculi
Orbicularis oris
Sternocleidomastoid
Trapezius
Deltoid
Pectoralis major
Biceps
Triceps
Latissimus dorsi
Rectus abdominis
Brachioradialis
Flexor carpi radialis

Internal oblique
Coracoid process
Deep muscles

Serratus posterior
Rhomboid major
Deep muscles
Teres

External oblique
Gluteus maximus
Sartorius
Biceps femoris - hamstrings
Rectus femoris - quadriceps
Semitendinosus - hamstrings
Gastrocnemius
Tibialis anticus
Achilles tendon

Erector spinae

Vastus medialis
Lateralis
Intermedius under Rectus femoris

Semimembranosus - hamstrings

This illustration shows the major muscles of the body and the fibrous sheaths that overlie them. Familiarity with the muscles and their location is essential for the masseur

BASICS

You may find the following guidelines helpful when you massage:

Warmth   One of your first considerations should be warmth. The room, the massage oil you use and your hands should all be warm. Cold temperatures make muscles contract, causing a loss of energy and feeling to both the giver and the receiver of the massage. Rub your hands together and make sure they are warm before you make contact. Keep the massage oil near a source of warmth such as a radiator. Place warm towels over the areas of the body you are not working on.

Clothing   As a masseur, wear loose-fitting clothes that give you freedom of movement. Natural fabrics such as cotton and linen are best as they allow your skin to breathe and are much more comfortable when you begin to get warmer.

Oils   There are many good massage oils, including coconut, sunflower, safflower and almond. Essential oils, which are also meant to have healing properties, are excellent. Olive oil is not recommended as it can stain clothing. Many of the massage oils sold at health shops are too heavily scented or too easily absorbed – test them before buying. Whatever you choose, it needs to be oil-based as other creams and lotions disappear into the skin too rapidly.

Where to massage   The most convenient and practical surface to use is the floor. Your partner should lie on a thin foam pad. This makes it easier to use your weight, direct energy and effort, do stretches and work Shiatsu points. When working on the floor, your movements will be slow, focused and well grounded.

   If you are massaging a number of people during the course of a day, it is better to use a massage table as you will not get so tired. A table is better for strokes as you are able to move easily alongside the body, varying the strokes and the areas you work on. The table needs to be low enough for you to lean your full body weight onto it.

Silent observation   It is better not to talk whilst you are giving a massage as you will be able to concentrate your energy more effectively. However, people sometimes talk because they are nervous and in such cases it will relax them. People also want to talk during massage because they are being emotionally affected by it. It is an excellent opportunity to work through psychological difficulties – you should direct the conversation to help them to open up. Whether you talk or not, it is important to observe closely your partner's breathing and watch out for any movement or change in the body or face. This will help you to see what effect you are having.

How deep?   Here you must trust your judgement and intuition. If an individual is physically strong and healthy, they will probably appreciate a deep treatment, whilst someone who is frail will probably want a softer one. Ideally, you should work as deeply as you can while staying just below the level of pain.

How long?   Massage treatments vary greatly in length. A general treatment lasts about 45 minutes to an hour and a half; specific injuries may take about 30 minutes, and work on headaches and neck tension may be even shorter. Whatever you are treating, trust your instincts to determine how long to work. A short, focused treatment can be as effective as a long one. You may lose concentration if you work for too long and this will diminish the effectiveness of the treatment.

Working the points   When you are manipulating the Shiatsu points, trust your intuition for finding the correct spot. If your partner feels you searching around and senses your uncertainty, they will become less relaxed and the treatment will be interrupted. You need to work with a directed confidence and your hands will soon learn.

When not to massage   You should not give a massage to anyone who has a serious illness and you should obviously avoid areas with serious injuries. Again, you must trust your intuition; work softly at first to see what kind of effect you are having. If you have any doubts – do not massage.

Intuition   I think it is worth emphasizing how important it is to learn to trust your intuition. Tune in to your own feelings about when and how to massage and finding the correct points to work. Use your own judgement and develop positions and movements to suit yourself and your partner.

As I am left-handed, some of you may find it awkward to follow the positioning exactly as in the photographs, but always work in a way that you find comfortable.

FUNDAMENTAL ENERGY

Energy is a basic concept of physics. Everything in the universe is made up of energy, from the most dense objects to the least – bones and blood, rocks and plant life and gases. The denser an object is, the less easily energy is able to flow through it. It is important that we become aware of our bodies as being more than just a physical structure of bones, tissue, blood, etc. Our vitality and our sense of aliveness come from energy; it shapes our individual natures and determines our relationships.

On a fundamental physical level we are composed of electromagnetic and electrochemical energy fields. These energy fields are in turn affected by the earth's magnetic fields, thereby linking us to the flow of energy around us.

Energy is the essence of everything; physical health and thus mental health and emotional well-being depend on it. It is the depth and substance of the subtle flow of energy within a body that determines the quality of that body's structure. It gives a person an expansive sense of presence and individuality that others can feel.

In this chapter, I want to explain my view of health, both physical and mental, and to explain how it can be achieved through massage and the various states of being involved in massage. It works as an introduction to the principles I base my work on.

BREATHING

Although fresh natural food and pure water are important sources of energy, breathing is the main source. The theory suggested by Ida Rolf and others is that breathing does not only supply the blood with oxygen via the lungs but that it is a nerve reflex. It directly stimulates the nerves along the spine, lengthening the spine and creating energy. Breath *is* energy. Learning to breathe correctly is therefore essential for our health and is also a vital tool in healing others.

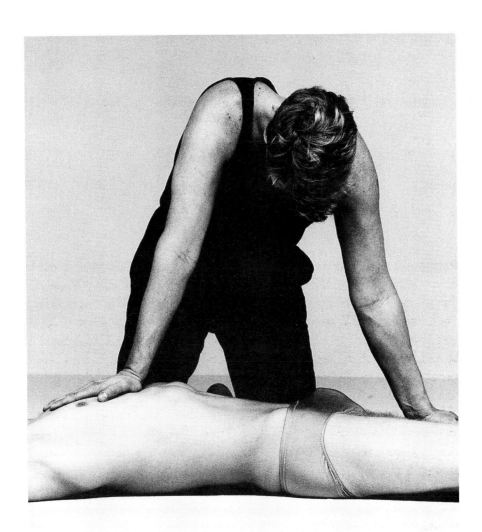

Maintain an awareness of your centre, or hara, while working

You should think of energy as being generated in *two* main places: in the thoracic and in the abdominal cavities. The thoracic cavity includes everything contained within the rib-cage, extending from the shoulders to the base of the ribs. The chest houses the body's two great pumps – the heart and the lungs. It draws in air to fuel the power centre of the lower body. The upper body is the centre of expression and vitality; the airy, expressive and conscious self.

The abdominal cavity is the area from just below the ribs and includes the whole pelvis region. The abdomen or belly is the centre where the body's power is generated. Rich with the fuel for life, it houses the organs controlling the metabolism, sex and digestion. The diaphragm, a large, dome-shaped muscle, separates the chest cavity from the abdominal cavity. If the diaphragm is relaxed, the breathing is able to move freely between the two centres.

Chest breathing, when the breathing is restricted to the thoracic cavity, is associated with physical activity and anxiety. When we do something physically strenuous or are frightened, the breathing naturally becomes rapid and shallow. Abdominal breathing, on the other hand, is deep and controlled and is associated with rest. It brings warmth and energy to the entire body. Deepening the capacity for energy in the lower centre opens up emotional feeling and generates power related to sexuality.

Containing and deepening   *Without working on ourselves, without developing our own inner life, we have nothing to give.* By working on the depth and quality of our breathing we increase our sensitivity to both receiving and transmitting energy. We need to become more conscious of the inner flow of energy connecting the mind and body, to concentrate on the movement of the breath, how it travels both downwards and upwards from the diaphragm. We should be able to feel how the air fills the two cavities. As concentration increases there will be a deepening feeling of personal power generated with each breath. We become more aware of the sense of space and clarity that breath creates, leaving us open to receive the flow of energy from other people. The regularity and depth of the breathing, and the containment of chi, in the form of air, within the body is a way of realizing our deepest and fullest potential for releasing and receiving energy.

CENTRING

When working with massage it is vital to maintain an awareness of your centre, your hara, the still place where movement and power are generated. It is a resting place, a centre of concentration and clarity, the beginning point for the cyclic path of energy. It gives time to receive information and process it. If you are correctly centred, if you can feel the breath filling your abdomen and the energy flowing to and from the hara, you will be able to work with openness, flexibility and strength.

GROUNDING

As you learn to feel your breath moving downwards and filling the abdominal cavity, it is important that you can also feel it extending around the cavity and into the back, and can sense your tailbone lengthening. This in turn brings energy into the legs and thus to the feet. As the energy flows downwards, you will, whilst standing still and quiet, feel your centre of gravity dropping. Your knees will relax and bend slightly and you will gain a sense of rootedness, of being 'grounded'. You should feel that you are squarely planted upon the ground, your weight should be evenly distributed, centred on your feet. To be well grounded your feet and legs must be strong, supple and relaxed.

This physical sense of grounding enables us to feel emotionally and psychologically secure. We are able physically to feel the inner self and its connection with the earth beneath us. With the weight of the body centred on the legs, we experience a sensation of emotional release and physical support. A secure sense of ground allows us first to identify and then release any tension in the body, tension that might otherwise interfere with the free flow of energy.

GIVING

A problem often encountered in massage is that of containing energy inside oneself and being unable to give. You should concentrate on maintaining an active stillness, on being positive and attentive, directing energy outwards with a sense of focus, and mentally visualizing the flow of energy inwards. Relax and concentrate. Learn to *feel* at a subtle level – to be able to give, you need to open up. Massage needs to move with the interplay of energy, both giving and receiving.

MASSAGE TECHNIQUES

The massage techniques I describe in this chapter will help you to learn to feel your energy as it flows around your body. They will also make you aware of your breathing patterns and your physicality – giving you the idea of your body as a connected whole.

While you are massaging, energy should flow from you through your hands. It is important to create space in your partner's body, to make it less dense, so that their energy can flow more easily. (You will begin to be able to recognize the texture of a body. If the muscles are well toned, there is a sense of fluidity within the tissue; they should be neither loose and weak nor tight and bound.)

You need to breathe deeply, lowering the breathing to the abdominal cavity. Because of the importance of deep breathing it is best if you work through the corrective relaxation exercises at the end of this chapter before starting on these movements. The simple, corrective breathing exercises are concerned with subtle mental and physical changes in both you and your partner and consequently are not always easy for beginners to grasp. (If you sense that your partner is finding them difficult, do not overdo it. If they go home with the knowledge you have given them and practise, the next treatment will be much easier.)

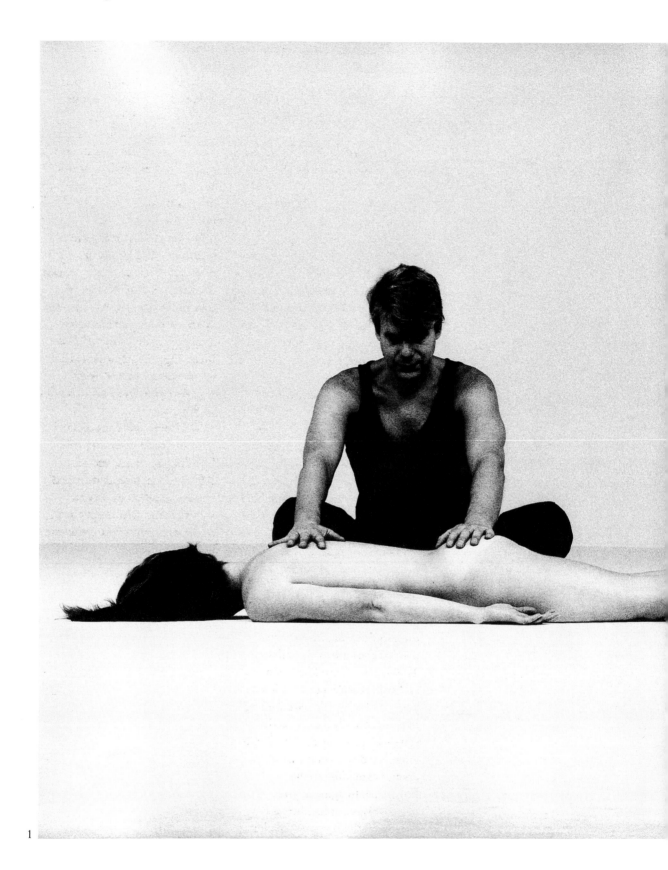

1

1. Balancing the energy of the back

This will help you to assess and, if need be, alter the breathing pattern of your partner. Small changes to breathing patterns can create change in the whole person.

Your partner should be lying on their front, with the head to one side and the arms lying loosely at the sides. Place yourself in line with the lower back, sitting comfortably on the floor. The initial physical contact is vital as it sets the mood for the entire treatment. You need to be aware of your inner body – your centre, your physical sense of ground and your breath. Turn your attention to your partner. Watch the breathing. Try to sense the energy flow and the general physical quality of your partner's body. Are there areas of tension? Are the joints strong and mobile? Is there a feeling of balance? Does the energy flow to the legs?

Make sure your hands are warm – if the environment is warm and your breath is deep, they will be. Place the right hand at the centre of the back, between the shoulder blades, and the left hand at the base of the tailbone. The contact should be positive and still, reaching out while also being receptive. You are seeking to achieve a relaxed, yet active, state – a 'quiet alert'. Your hands are relaxed and warm, with energy extending to the fingertips. Imagine in your mind's eye your hands making contact with your partner's inner body beneath the surface of the skin.

Keep your shoulders open, not hunched, and focus all your energy upon your partner. Synchronize your breathing with that of your partner. If theirs is rapid and shallow, follow suit. Your intention is to become part of your partner's body, to blend imperceptibly with it.

If your partner has been breathing rapidly and shallowly, now is the time to start a process of change. Subtly deepen your own breath so that, having been synchronized, you are now drawing attention to a different breathing pattern, which your partner, as a result of your concentration and sensitivity, will respond to.

Maintain your awareness of your own and your partner's breathing patterns, and of differences in temperature and texture, at all times. Try to stimulate the cold, empty areas, to instil energy, and to relax the hot areas.

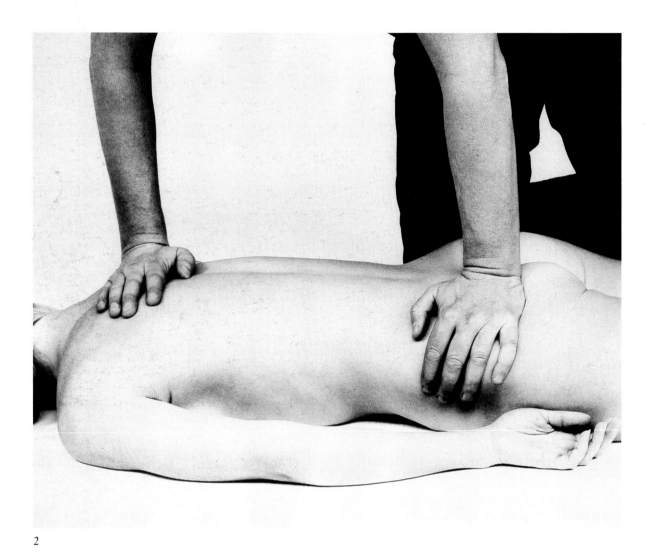

2

2. Balancing the structure of the back

The idea in this series of movements is to learn to use the weight of your body and your strength in an efficient and focused, rather than generalized, fashion; to stretch out and relax your partner's body in diagonal directions across the spine.

Kneel next to your partner and place one hand on your partner's left hip and the other on their opposite shoulder. Bend your knees and lean your weight equally between both arms. Your elbows should be slightly bent, allowing your shoulders and arms to relax – the effort should come from the weight of your body. The lower you bend your knees and the more you lean and focus your weight between your arms,

the greater the stretch. Feel your partner's body being stretched in opposition across the spine.

Next, stretch the right hip and left shoulder. Then, stretch out the hip and shoulder of one side, followed by the hip and shoulder of the other.

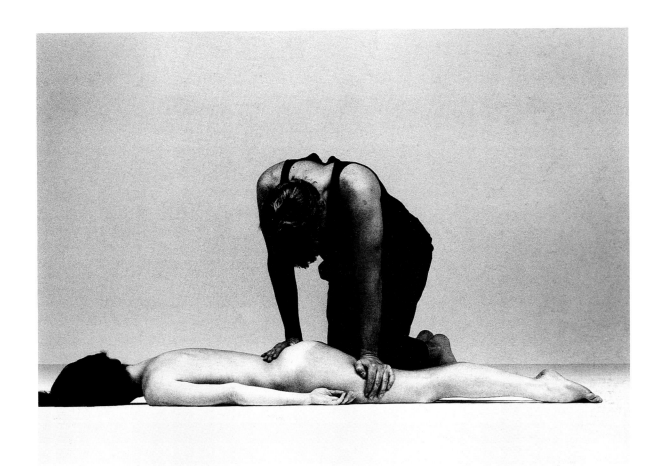

3

3. Opposition stretch from pelvis to thigh

This stretch opens the hip joint and increases the sense of connection between the legs and the main structure of the body.

Standing or kneeling and leaning over your partner, place one hand on the hip nearest you and the other hand on the opposite thigh. If standing, bend your knees, then centre your weight between your arms and lean.

Change to the other hip and opposite thigh, and then work the hip and leg of the same side together, followed by the hip and leg of the other side.

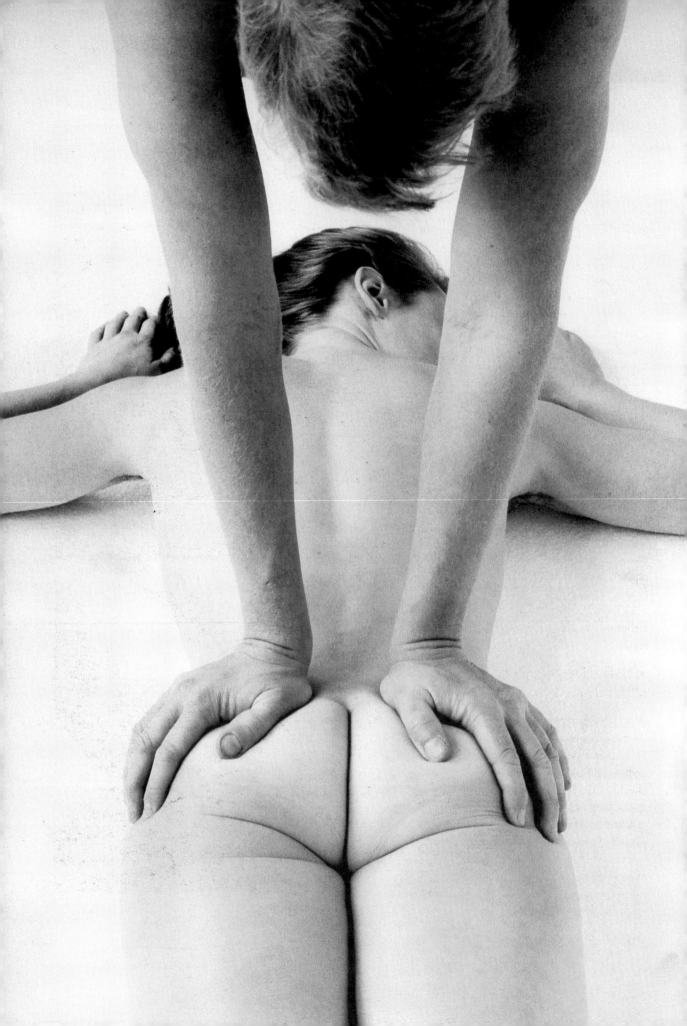

4. Directing energy down the back

A dense, rounded back indicates an over-activity of energy directed upwards at the back. Tension is often held deep within the body without our being consciously aware of it; it becomes a part of our personal image. This technique aims to redirect the energy so that it flows up the front of the body and down the back.

a) Kneel at your partner's head – they should still be lying on their front – and place your hands on their shoulders. Direct your weight and energy down the back; try to visualize the energy flowing from your centre, through your hands and down your partner's back. (See the illustration on p. 42.)

b) Then move your hands to the rounded upper back and again lean your weight towards the feet and focus your attention on feeling the energy.

c) Finally, move your hands to either side of the pelvis and repeat.

5. Balancing the energy of the front

With your partner now lying on their back, observe the breathing pattern and the two breathing centres: the abdomen and the chest cavities. The longer you spend watching, the more you will see. The front is more revealing as it is softer and more vulnerable than the back. It is also easier for your partner to breathe in this position.

a) Place your warm, energized hands on the two centres. Concentrate on the breathing, synchronize your own with your partner's. Use your intuition as you work. Make subtle changes in your own breathing pattern or give verbal suggestions to encourage your partner to deepen and soften their breathing. Try to make your partner aware of the things you observe.

b) Move one or both of your hands to other areas – the head, legs, feet – in order to develop a sense of feel. (See, for example, the illustration on p. 19.) Sense how cool the legs can be in relation to the forehead, which is often over-active with thought.

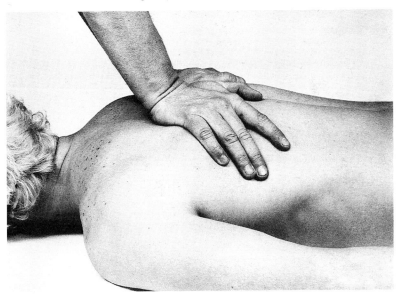

4b

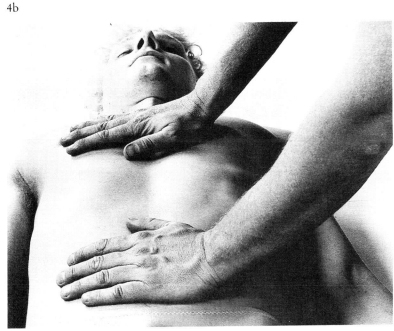

5a

4c

6. Balancing the structure of the front

With these movements you are working to open all the joints in the body. As you did with the back, use the weight and position of your body to correct the alignment of your partner's body.

a) Kneeling beside your partner – they should be lying on their back – place your hands on the right shoulder and left hip and lean your body weight evenly. Then change to the left shoulder and right hip. Then work the shoulder and hip of the same side, and of the other side. This will stretch your partner's body, giving a feeling of release. You will find that alternately leaning and releasing using a rocking movement will help to relax both you and your partner.

b) Release tightly held and tense thighs by standing at their feet and putting a hand on each thigh. Lean with your weight to open the thighs outwards. (See the top illustration on p. 78.) You can also use a stretching movement, placing one hand on the thigh and the other on the opposite hip bone, to widen the space between the hip and pelvis. (See the top illustration on p. 81.)

c) Kneeling at your partner's head, place your hands on the shoulders and lean your weight downwards.

d) Then, crouching and grasping your partner's arms just above the wrist and pulling the arms back and away from the body, lean your weight back to lengthen the upper body.

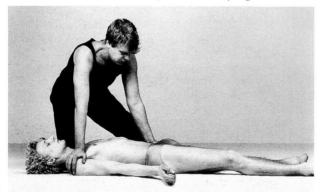

6a

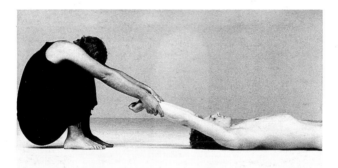

6d

7. Pulling the legs

This stretch will release the tension in the joints of the ankles, knees and hips.

Stand or sit at your partner's feet, hold the feet and lean back, using your weight to release the hip joints. Stretch both legs together.

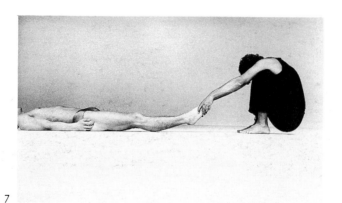

7

6c

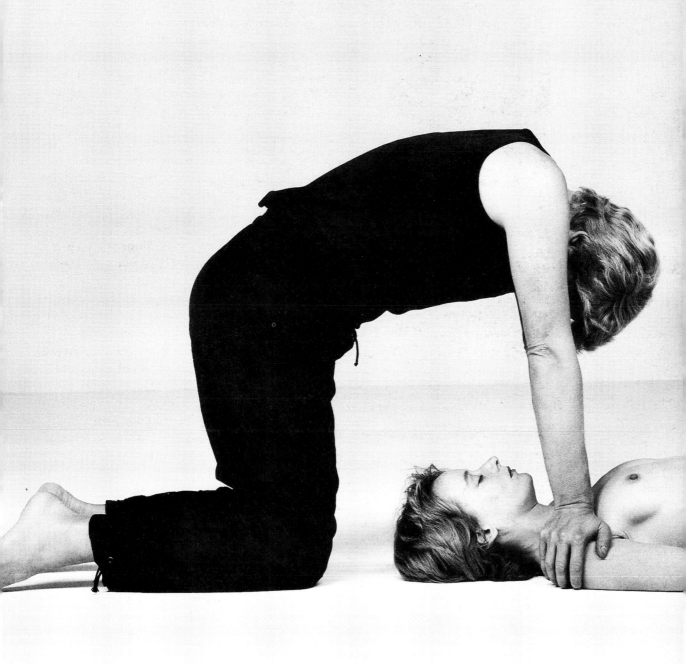

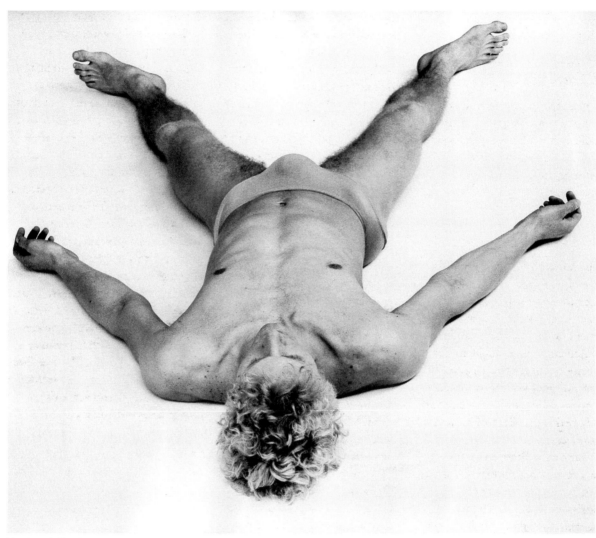

Ex 1 and Ex 2

FUNDAMENTAL CORRECTIVE RELAXATION EXERCISES

You and your partner can do these exercises together. They will teach you about your body and enable you to centre yourself, learning the value of deep breathing.

Exercise 1

The more time you give to this exercise in passive observation, the more you will learn about your own body. Focusing your attention on your body and its alignment whilst you lie in this position will give you a good indication of your posture when standing. You will be able to feel where there is a lack of balance or connection.

Lie on the floor on your back in a comfortable position. Close your eyes. Sense your body's position, its weight and its relation to the ground. You need to 'give in' completely to the ground in order to become aware of the subtle feelings within yourself. Concentrate entirely on each part of your body, focusing your attention on your joints, the points of connection in your body. Visualize the spaces between the joints which give a sense of openness and length to the body. Imagine that your body is moving as you lie there motionlessly. Does your body feel balanced and aligned? Is one shoulder higher than the other, one leg longer, or one hip joint tighter? Are your thighs open and relaxed? As you visualize this subtle sense of movement in your body you will begin to feel the pull of the various imbalances increasing. A high left shoulder will begin to feel even tighter, while the opposing short right leg will feel shorter. As you become more aware of a tight hip joint it may even begin to ache.

Exercise 2

This exercise is designed for you to become aware of your breathing, to be able to direct your breath to different parts of the body. As you do this you will become aware of areas of tension in your body. To be able to feel your breath in a tight, dense part of the body is the first step to releasing it. Learning to experience your body in this way will help you to explore your innermost feelings.

Place yourself comfortably on the floor, lying on your back. Concentrate on your breathing and just be with it. There is no need to do anything. Sense if the breath is deep and balanced between the two centres – the abdomen and chest. Visualize your inner body; focus on the vital organs, one by one; sense their function and quality. Feel the breath, your energy, washing over each individual organ, calming and revitalizing it.

Relax your chest and direct your breathing into your abdomen. Visualize the breath travelling down into the hips and lengthening the tailbone. The exhalation is important; make sure that all the breath goes out. When the abdomen is empty of breath, pause, until there is a natural impulse to breath in again. Your chest should be passive while you work to develop depth in your breathing and a sense of connection in your lower body, warming and calming the vital organs of the abdomen.

After a few minutes, reverse the flow of breath. Take breath into the chest, whilst allowing the abdomen to remain passive. The breathing should be deep and relaxed. Sense the breath as it extends out towards the sides and back, filling the entire rib-cage. If you have tight, 'held' shoulders and neck, you will begin to feel the breath in them. The free flow of breath, of energy, is essential in this area as the upper body expresses our vitality.

THE BACK AND SHOULDERS

The back, with the spine as its central pole, can be seen as a mirror image of our general health. Our ability to cope with everyday stress, the functioning of our essential organs, the health of our nervous system – all depend on the vitality of the spine. The state we are trying to achieve with the spine is lengthened, flexible balance.

The spine, or spinal column, comprises 24 small bones, or true vertebrae. There are seven cervical vertebrae, twelve thoracic and five lumbar vertebrae. Each vertebra is separated from the next by a spinal disc. These intervertebral discs are elastic in nature, facilitating the mobility of the back. They act as shock absorbers when the back is jolted, as it is, for example, whenever we walk or run. Stretchy ligaments connect the 24 vertebrae to one another. The spine is stabilized by powerful muscles connected to the vertebrae, the back of the chest wall and the pelvis. The structure can easily be visualized by imagining the spine as a mast held in place by stays in the form of muscles.

If you look at yourself in profile in the mirror, you will see that the spine shows a series of natural curves which are designed to allow, in a healthy person, the maximum movement, flexibility and strength. It is only if these curves become extremely exaggerated that they present a problem, imposing increased strain on the back.

During training, dancers learn to work with the concept of lifting from the ears, stretching the spine against the opposing weight of the pelvis. Lifting like this, it is as if they are trying to take the curve out of the spine. The result is to make it easier for the body to balance on the skeletal structure, thus freeing the muscles from postural support and allowing them to carry out their main task of movement. This idea is used in most corrective posture work, particularly the Alexander technique. Ida Rolf also uses a similar concept with her image of a 'sky hook' lifting the body from the top of the head.

The problems encountered by the spine stem from its vertical position. Since mankind began walking upright, thousands of years ago, the spine has had to work in constant opposition to the pull of gravity. It has the intricate task of balancing the opposing weight of the rib-cage, the shoulders and arms, and the head and neck, through an infinite range of movements and weight changes – a task made more complicated by the fact that we are in a state of constant, although sometimes very subtle, motion. When the spine is stretched and the body is 'lifted', an efficient, fluid relationship with gravity is easier. This efficiency is almost impossible for people with bad posture, whose shoulders are 'held', tense and rigid.

The major muscle group affecting movement of the spine is the erector spinae. These muscles extend the full length of the spine on both sides. They are thick at the lower back and split into thin bundles on their way towards the head, securing attachments to the ribs, upper vertebrae and neck. The shoulder girdle, which consists of the clavicle, or collar bone, and the scapula, or shoulder blade (a large, flat bone), balances delicately on the upper part of the skeletal structure. Its only bony attachment to the trunk is the point where the clavicle joins the top of the sternum. The scapula is connected to the spine, from the middle of the back to the neck, by muscles including the trapezius, which is flat and wide. As its only connection to the spine is muscular, the scapula thus has potential for extreme freedom of movement. The muscles of the shoulder are thin, flat and interwoven with one another. When misused they tangle into 'knots', causing stiffness and a limited range of movement.

According to Shiatsu theory, the back contains the major meridian of the body's 12 energy pathways. This is the bladder meridian, which runs the full length of the spine, on both sides of it, on its way from the neck down the back of the legs to the feet. It is the longest meridian in the body and affects all the other meridians. The acupressure points on the bladder meridian along the back stimulate spinal nerves connected to all the body's organs. The points at the upper back stimulate the lungs and heart and can be used to combat colds, breathing difficulties, insomnia, emotional problems and general stress. Points further down the back can be worked to stimulate the digestion, and lower still, in the lumbar area, are the points affecting elimination of the body's waste products. With training one can use these points to diagnose the condition of the organs.

The gall bladder meridian runs along the top of each shoulder and into the back of the skull. Points along it can be worked to help alleviate colds, headaches, mental stress and stiff shoulders. Part of the small intestine meridian crosses the centre of the scapula and this too can be stimulated to help reduce stress and stiffness in the shoulders.

In our head-dominated, stressful, Western culture the tendency is to draw an excess of energy into the upper back, neck and shoulders. This causes stiffness, hypertension (high blood pressure), migraines and flu. You can learn a great deal about your own body from looking around you. Watch someone in a repetitive activity such as jogging, especially as they are getting tired and having to exert themselves. The head stretches forward, the chest sticks out, while the shoulders and arms go up and out to the sides. Notice how the upper body takes on the work of the lower body. The chest becomes the power centre when in fact the power needs to come from below. It is will and determination that drives them and not the strong, fluid power from below. If you were to feel the jogger's back, you would feel heat, a bound density between the shoulder blades and a cold emptiness in the lower back.

Problems in the back also develop from the lack of physical and psychological energy that comes with ageing. The body compresses and thickens – taking on the look of 'middle-aged spread'.

To avoid all these problems we must change the bad movement habits that have developed from years of misusing our bodies. Many of these start in childhood, as a result of bad physical training; even the transition from crawling to walking is vitally important. We tend to want to put a baby on its feet too early rather than letting it go through the intricate process of opposition reach and pull, of finding its own feet. All through our lives we take lazy shortcuts to reach the goal quickly, when in reality the process is the goal.

MASSAGE TECHNIQUES

The back is a good place to begin a complete massage treatment. It is best to use a variety of movements. Interplay pressure on deep trigger points with soothing strokes, and movements which cover the whole back with ones that concentrate on more specific areas. Always work anatomically correctly, in line with the direction of the muscles *or* directly across them. Do not place direct pressure on the spine except with the flat hand for the long, balancing stretch of technique 3. Pay attention to your partner's breathing pattern throughout, as changes and reactions are less obvious on the back.

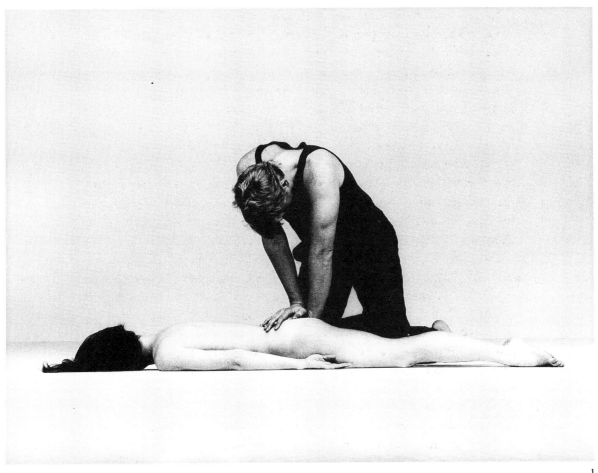

1

1. Stretching the tailbone

This is designed to release tension in the lower back, to correct posture-related problems such as the pelvis tilting forward, the stomach sagging and the buttocks sticking out, and bladder and sexual problems caused by tension and withholding.

Kneel next to your partner, in line with the buttocks and place yourself well above the sacrum, the large wedge-shaped bone in the lower part of the back. With your arms extended, but not locked, and the heel of the left hand pointing towards the feet, place your right hand over your left and push the tailbone straight down towards the floor. The further your hands slide down over the edge of the tailbone, the greater the stretch, and thus the greater the release of tension.

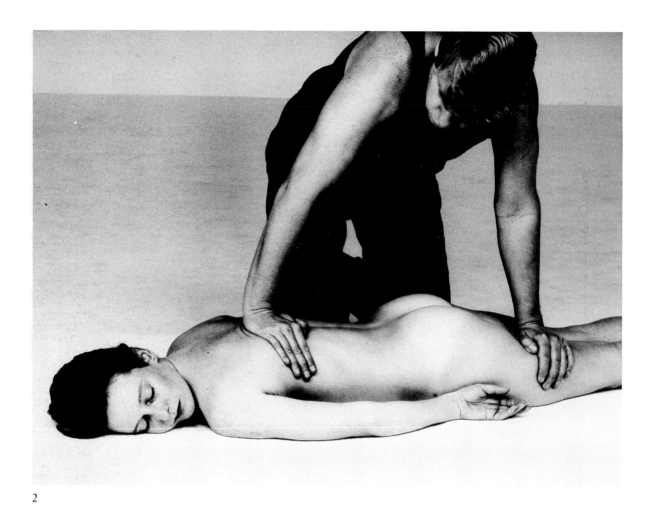

2

2. Balancing the erector spinae muscles

This is intended to bring resilience and balance to the major muscle group affecting the spine. It helps to move stagnant body fluids towards the heart by stimulating the circulation of the blood and the lymph. You will be working on the major Shiatsu meridian, the bladder meridian, and this will benefit the vital organs. The movement also alleviates back pain.

Beginning in the same position as the previous movement, place your left hand on the centre of your partner's left thigh, well above the knee. (You should never apply pressure directly on or behind the knee.) Place your right hand just to the left of the base of the spine, with the heel of your hand on the erector spinae muscle. Leaning your weight onto your hand, stroke the full length of the muscle, taking care to follow through around the shoulder. By moving your body

and shifting your weight so that it is centred over your arm as you slide up the back, you will maintain a deep, even pressure throughout the full length of the stroke. Be sure to keep your hand relaxed with the fingers lying flat so that you are massaging with the whole of your hand. Work both sides of the spine several times.

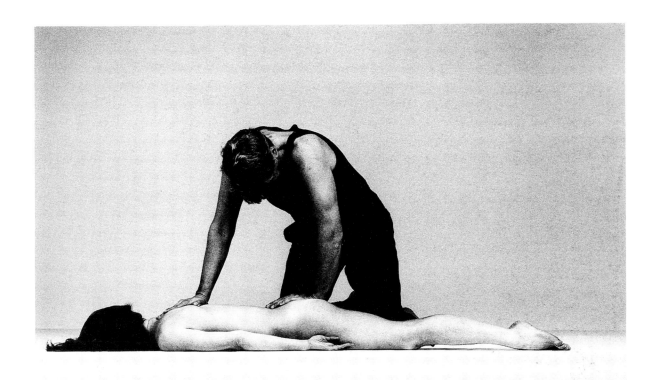

3a

3. Balancing the back

a) Kneel next to your partner close to the centre of the back. Place your left hand on the centre of the sacrum and the right hand on the middle of the upper back. Lean your weight first onto one arm, then the other, so that you can feel your partner's spine lengthen.

b) Move your left hand to the left side of the sacrum and place your right hand on the upper back to the right of the spine. Again lean your weight onto your hands so that the stretch goes across the spine. You can add a rocking motion as it is relaxing and will help to free tight vertebrae. Do both sides. (See the illustration on p. 24.)

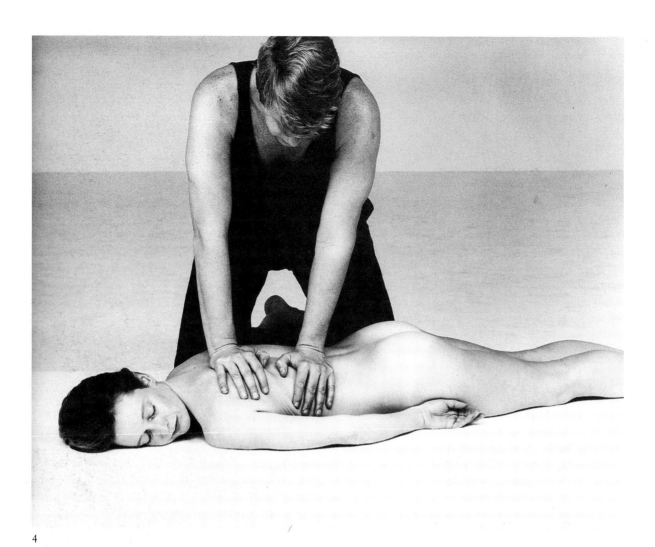

4

4. Creating space between the muscle and the spine

As well as the rounding and shortening of the spine caused by the downward pull of gravity on a poorly aligned body, the spine is sometimes pulled to one side causing an uneven development of the erector muscles. Either way, the often severe curves in the spine leave the lower and upper back weak, causing compression of the vertebrae and a humped tensing of the muscles at the centre of the back. We need to open the space between the erector muscles and the spine which will alleviate the stress caused by this condition and will 'suggest' to the nervous system a more correct posture.

From a kneeling position at the centre of the back, reach across the spine and place the heels of both hands in the space between the large band of erector muscles and the spine at the point where the back humps. If there is too little space, the muscle is over-developed and tight; too much space, and the muscle is weak.

Try to develop a sense of what a well-toned muscle feels like. With your heels in the space, push into and over the muscle, continuing over the ribs to the floor. For deeper penetration, use your thumbs.

To release stress along the whole of the vulnerable upper spine, you can run your thumbs from the same starting point all along the edge of the spine and the erector muscles, taking the movement up and around the shoulder.

5. Freeing the scapulae

The scapula is attached to the spine by muscle, giving it the potential for extreme freedom of movement. Unfortunately it does not always work that way in reality. Heavy physical work and stress-forming activities often result in the shoulders tightening up and being held high and rounded. This technique should help to loosen them.

Kneeling next to your partner's left shoulder blade, with their head turned away from you, lift the left arm and place the forearm across the back. Place your left hand under the shoulder, your arm supporting the arm, and gently lift. From this position you can perform several manipulations.

a) With your right hand, trace around and under the inner edges of the shoulder blades, using the web between your thumb and first finger placed flat over the back.

b) You can also use your thumb or fingers to probe deeply under the blade.

Rotating the shoulder by moving your left arm in a small, circular motion is also effective.

Repeat all the movements with the right shoulder blade, kneeling on your partner's right side.

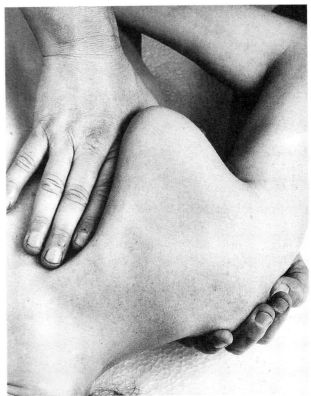

5a

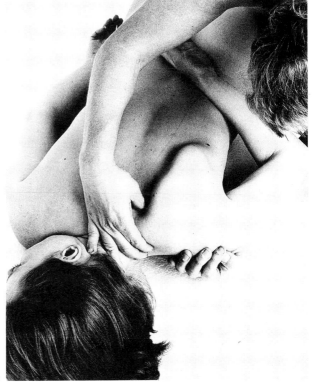

5b

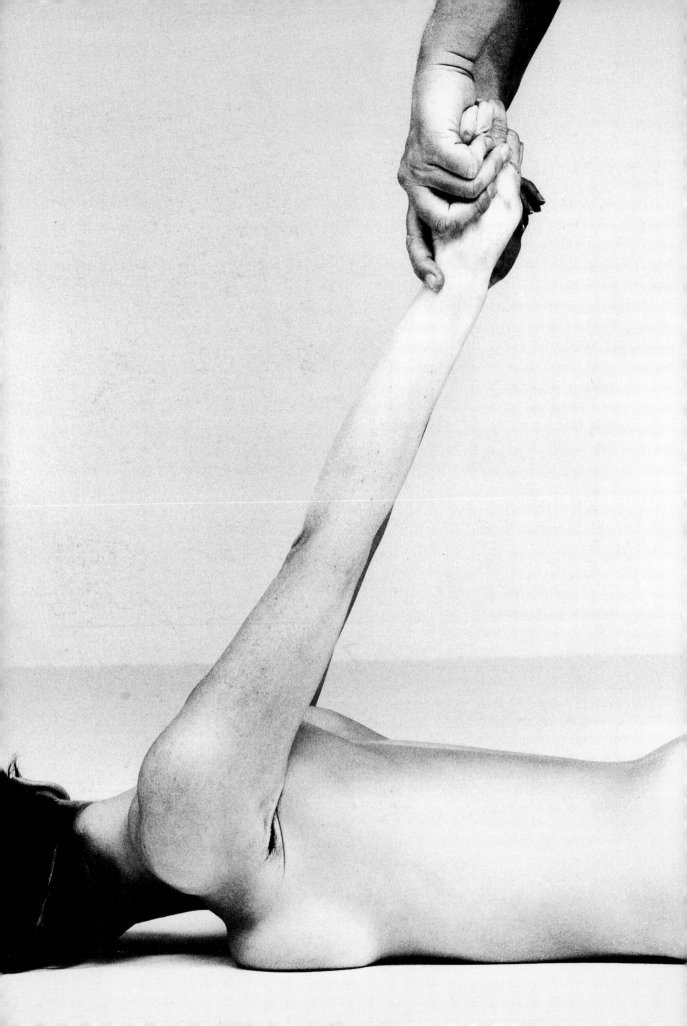

6. Stretching the shoulders

This is a good stretch for freeing stiff shoulders.

From a standing position, grasp your partner's hands and slowly and carefully lift the arms up and back. Most people's arms will not extend back as far as the dancer's shown in the illustration, so take care.

7. Squeezing the neck

This is designed to smoothe away tiredness from the muscles of the neck.

Lying with their face to the floor, your partner may want to put a hand beneath their forehead. Cup your hands around the back of the neck, squeezing and working out the tension. The deeper you can cup your hands around, and into, the neck, the better. Take the movement well into the base of the skull and down to the shoulder. You will find that squeezing the large trapezius muscles that extend from the neck to the shoulder is also effective.

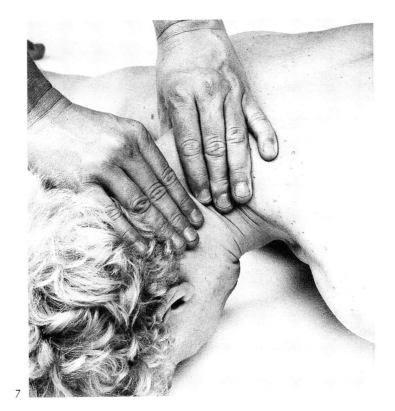

7

8. Stimulating the base of the skull

The area at the base of the skull contains important points which can be worked to give relief from headaches and general tension.

With your partner in the same position on the floor, use the fingers (one on top of the other) or the thumb of one hand to probe around the base of the skull, stimulating the points where the muscles are attached at the base.

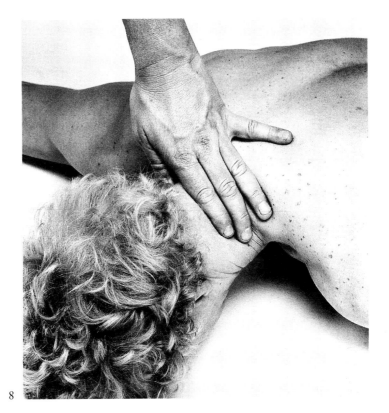

8

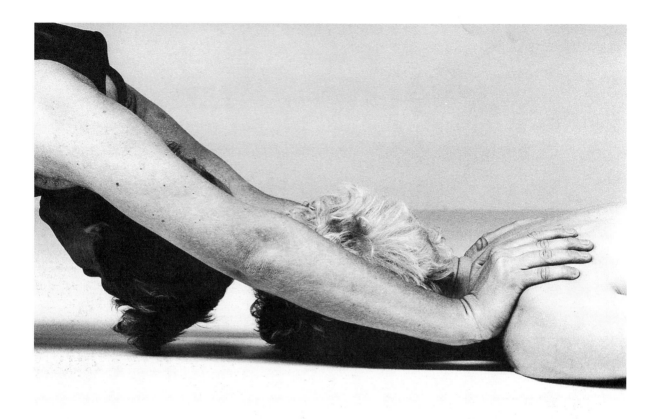

9

9. Grounding and directing the shoulders down

The preceding strokes were concerned mostly with moving stagnant, trapped fluids and revitalizing muscle tissue by stimulating blood flow to the heart. The following four techniques work down the body to focus concentration and ground the energy.

The thumbs become important as tools to trigger points related to specific organs. Do not worry about being exactly on a point. Trust your hands; work with a focused confidence and you will be in the right place.

Kneel at your partner's head, well back from it, keeping low and in line with your partner's body. Place a hand on each shoulder, extend your arms, lengthen your back and simply lean your weight into their shoulders, directing them towards the floor. Hold this pose for about 10 or 15 seconds and release. Repeat this a couple of times.

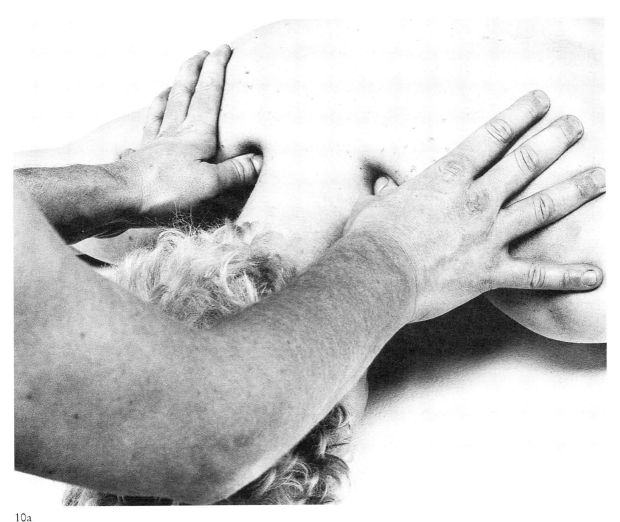

10a

10. Shoulder Shiatsu

a) Kneel directly in front of your partner's head. Use a subtle shift of weight to direct your thumbs along the gall bladder meridian, which lies along the top of the shoulders. Remember to keep close to the floor and in line with your partner's body, so that you can almost feel the continuous stream of energy flowing along your spine and into your partner.

b) Still kneeling, draw yourself up so that you are directly over the head. Using your thumbs, stimulate the small intestine point in the centre of each scapula, working directly down towards the floor. Trust your hands to find where the points are.

10b

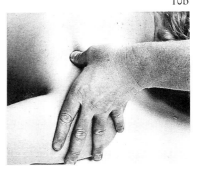

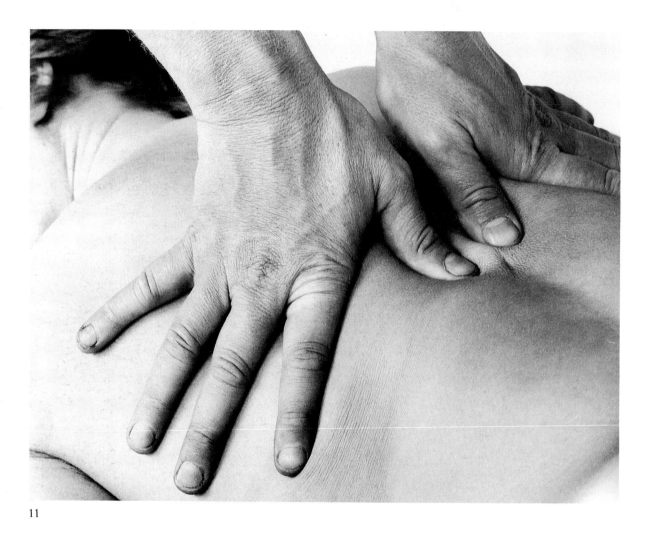

11

11. Working the bladder meridian

The chief meridian of the body, the bladder meridian, is located close to the spine.

Rise up on your knees, extending your arms from above, and work the points along both sides of the spine with your thumbs. Start from between the shoulder blades and work down to the bladder points on the sacrum (see the illustration on pp. 54-5). If you find any sore spots, go back and work them again.

12. Soft finishing strokes

To complete the massage of the back, stroke the erector muscles on either side of the spine with the heel of each hand from a kneeling position at the head, grounding and balancing energy along the length of the back. Let the heels of your hands trace the ridge of the pelvis down to the floor. Then draw back along the spine with a stroke directed towards the shoulders. Repeat this series of strokes several times.

Be sure to use your weight and push into the pelvis to stretch the lower back. If you wish to direct more weight, and therefore more stretch, into your partner's lower back, come up off your knees onto your feet, so that most of your weight is now behind your arms.

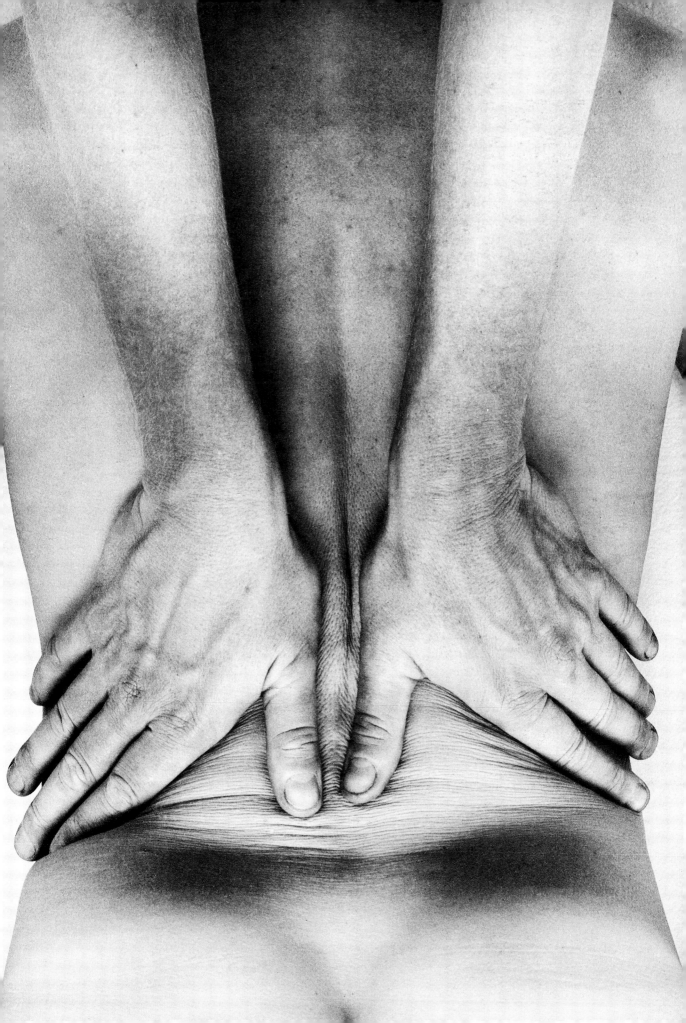

CORRECTIVE RELAXATION EXERCISES

You can do these exercises to relieve tensions in the back and reduce stress. Like all the corrective relaxation exercises in this book, they are for both you and your partner, to do whenever you feel they may be useful.

Exercise 1

This is a good exercise for increasing the flexibility of the spine. It opens and releases tension in the chest and deepens the breathing.

Sit back to back with your partner on the floor, making sure that your lower backs are pushed together. Most people's legs will not be as flexible as these dancers', so sit with your legs in a comfortable position. Take a few minutes to relax and concentrate on synchonizing your breathing with your partner's. The breath should be directed downwards. On the inhalation you will feel the base of your backs pushing against each other. On one of the out breaths, you should push back as your partner yields. Complete the exhalation, pushing gently with your body weight. As the movement comes to a natural finish, your partner will push back to the upright poisition on the inhalation and continue pushing as you both breathe out. Repeat this several times, remaining conscious of your breathing. Keep your lower backs in contact and the breathing directed downwards.

I use this exercise in massage classes to teach how to give weight, to feel the legs as a source of both power and of connection to the ground. It relaxes, centres and balances the body.

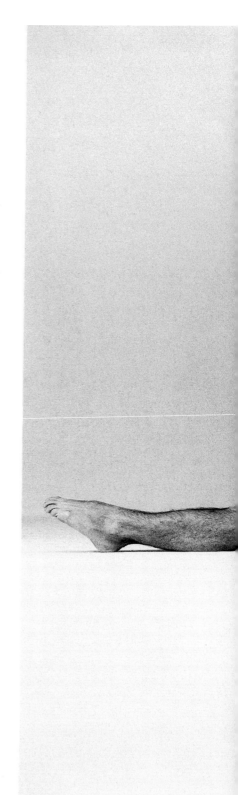

Ex 1

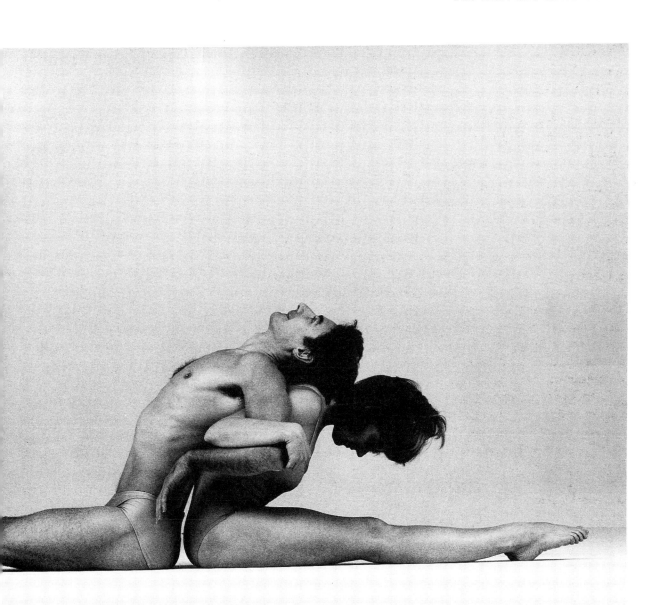

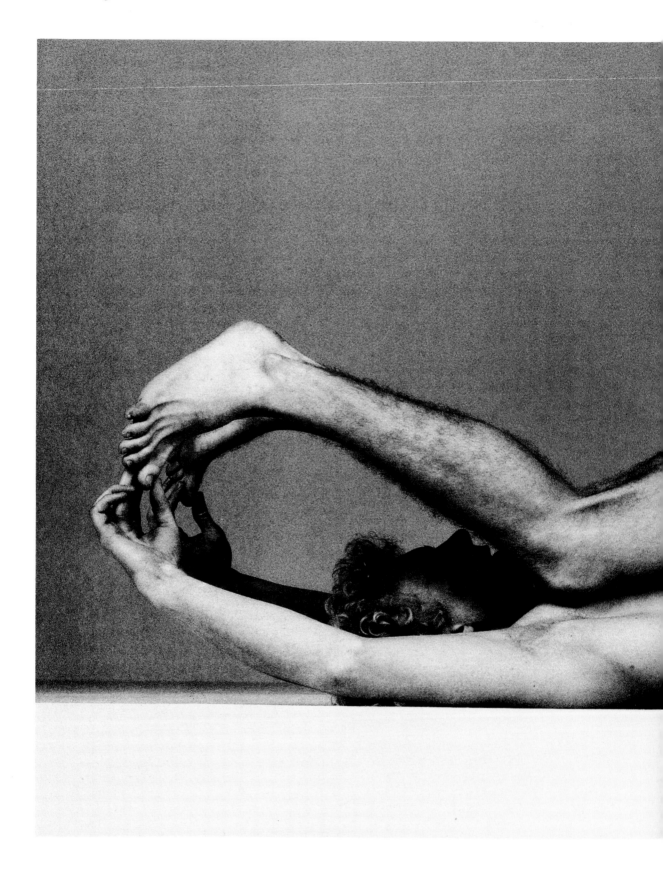

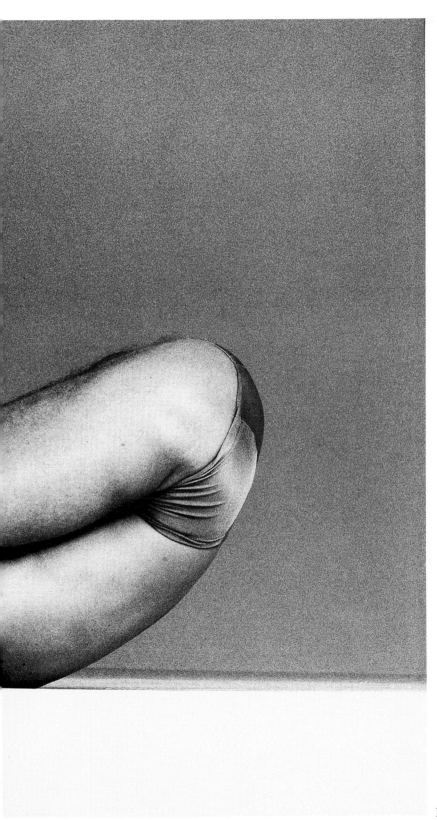

Exercise 2

This exercise is designed to stretch the lower back and develop its mobility. It will help you to feel the connection between the pelvis and the lower back, strengthening the muscles of the lower back which extend all the way into the pelvis. The pelvis is often tilted forwards, thus weakening these muscles.

Lie on your back on the floor and clasp your knees to your chest. Concentrate on your breathing and regulate it so that it is deep and even.

Now direct the thrust of your central body weight and energy down into the floor so that the buttocks and tailbone come up and your legs extend up over your face. Reach out and clasp your toes to retain your balance. Sense the opposing pulls of gravity.

Ex 2

THE PELVIS
AND BACK OF THIGHS

The pelvic cavity forms an essential connection between the expressive, fluid energy and vitality of the upper body and the supportive, power-generating and grounding energy of the legs. The bowl-shaped pelvis sits firmly secured in a central position in the body, giving it balanced strength. Its role is to house and protect the abdominal organs and to transfer weight from the upper body to the lower limbs. The pelvis is also an attachment point for many muscles that are important for the balance, movement and stability of the entire body.

The pelvis is essentially a firm ring of bone made up of two hip bones, with the tailbone, or sacrum, at the centre. Each individual hip bone is formed from a fusion of three bones: the ilium, the ischium and the pubis. The wedge-shaped sacrum acts as a keystone and support to the spine as it secures the two hip bones to the vertically balanced spine at the fifth lumbar vertebra. This point is called the lumbrosacral joint.

Sacrum means sacred bone; in Buddhism the sacrum is thought to house the body's fundamental energy. The pelvis is the physical centre of the emotions, of sexuality and fertility, as it houses the reproductive organs and their outlets. Although it varies with different bodies, the lumbrosacral joint is generally considered to be the body's centre of gravity – the divine neutral point where movement and energy are generated, the hara. In the disciplines of the martial arts, it is considered a central point of concentration on the way to attaining spiritual and physical strength. To live in the body, you need to experience the centre, the body's mind. It is also the point where you first experience the physical sensation of gravity's natural pull downwards.

Ida Rolf's image of lifting a slumped body off the ground by securing a hook to the centre of the head is useful in understanding our relation to gravity. The spine would be lengthened by the opposing pull of the pelvis, and the weight of the legs would open spaces within the compressed thigh, knee and ankle joints. With the body placed on the ground, the anti-gravity muscles of the calf, the front of the thigh and the buttocks need to be strong and flexible in order to maintain a similarly balanced, upright alignment. Unfortunately, ageing, lack of regular exercise and poor postural habits weaken these muscles, and the entire body suffers a diminishment of strength and mobility. Over-tight muscles, caused by incorrect and repetitive exercise, can have the same effect; muscles need to be elastic and fluid. The hamstrings are an example of a muscle group that easily become over-developed – they often thicken and glue together. When the hamstrings are too tight they pull, compress and tilt the pelvis, and can cause pain at the knees.

The classic image of the 'beer belly' is more often a problem of posture than weight. The organs are spilled from their container as the belly is thrust forward and the spine curves severely inwards in the lumbrosacral area. This weakens the connection through the pelvis to the thighs and inhibits the spinal nerves, adversely affecting the digestive organs and kidneys. The diaphragm is also affected, and breathing is restricted. The loss of connection to the legs leaves the thigh joints weak and compressed: the weight is loaded hard onto the front of the joints. These imbalances are often further aggravated by the legs and feet turning out in a bid to regain stability, which naturally restricts movement. Can you imagine a car moving forward with its wheels turned out?

Ideally, the leg muscles should be elastic, strong and well balanced. The joints need to be aligned and supported by the deep muscles and the ligaments. The feet should be parallel, in the forward direction we want to move. Being grounded properly, drawing the body's energy downwards, gives greater control and power to our fundamental physical and emotional energy. If you watch an animal that moves on all fours, it is easy to see power coming from the hind legs, while the focus and direction of movement extends through the spine to the head. Watch someone throwing a ball to see how power and control come from the lower part of the body; not merely from the arm but from the thigh and pelvis. The lower you can take the centre of gravity, the greater the control and power.

MASSAGE TECHNIQUES

The main points to bear in mind when working on the pelvis and thighs are their functions of physical support and of connecting the upper body with the lower. Try to visualize and understand the transfer of weight downwards, and of power upwards, through the pelvis, and the openness within the pelvis and thighs in relation to emotional energy. You will be working on lengthening the legs and creating space between compressed joints. Pay particular attention to the alignment of the pelvis and the hips and all the muscles of the buttocks, thighs and calves.

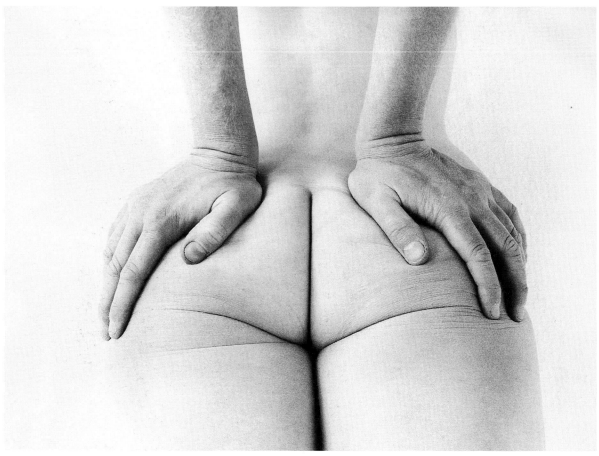

2a

1. Stretching the tailbone

This movement helps to stimulate the flow of fundamental energy upwards through the body. As a result of wrongly developed or weak muscles, the top of the pelvis is often tilted forwards, adversely affecting the postural integrity of the body, the organs of digestion, the kidneys, the adrenal gland and the breathing. This stretch will help to alleviate these problems and also relax tension in the pelvis area, particularly tension caused by anger and sexually related fear. The sacrum is associated with both these emotions.

Kneel next to your partner, in line with their buttocks so that you are placed just past the end of the tailbone. Put your left hand on the sacrum, directing the heel of the hand towards your partner's feet. Place your right hand over your left. As you breathe out, lean your relaxed weight down towards the floor. You should feel the pelvis tilting. Although the pelvis is strong, the sacrum is sensitive, so do the movement with care. Focus your attention, the weight of your body and your breathing. Always keep a clear image in your mind of what you are trying to do and visualize yourself going through the movement. You can add a rocking movement to help with relaxing and opening the pelvis.

This stretch is the same as the tailbone stretch in the lesson on the back (see the illustration on p. 35). I repeat it here because it is such an important one.

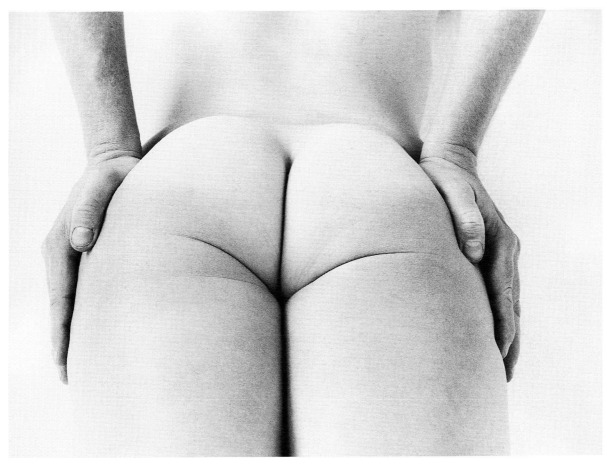

2b

2. Releasing compressed vertebrae of the lower spine

This technique is intended to release any compressed vertebrae in the lower back and sacrum area. The condition often arises as a consequence of a poor, slumping posture which causes the body's weight to be directed onto the small of the back. You are seeking to relax the tight muscles of the lower back and to relieve any pain in the sciatic nerve (which runs from the lower hip to the calf). Any sexual or emotional problems of a physical origin should also be helped with this technique.

a) Stand at your partner's head and place your hands on both sides of the sacrum. Lean your weight towards your partner's feet. Hold the position at first as a stretch, release, then stretch again a few times with a rocking movement.

b) Repeat the movement with your hands a little further apart.

3. Working the bladder points

You are now working the acupressure points along the bladder meridian as a deeper stimulus. Working the bladder meridian is particularly useful in resolving pelvic and bladder problems.

Place yourself close to your partner's sacrum and use both thumbs to work the points along the edge of the sacrum on both sides. Be sure that the effort comes from your centre and not just from your hands and arms. Use your energy, with the help of deep controlled breathing, right from your feet through your body to achieve powerful pressure. (See the illustration on the following page.)

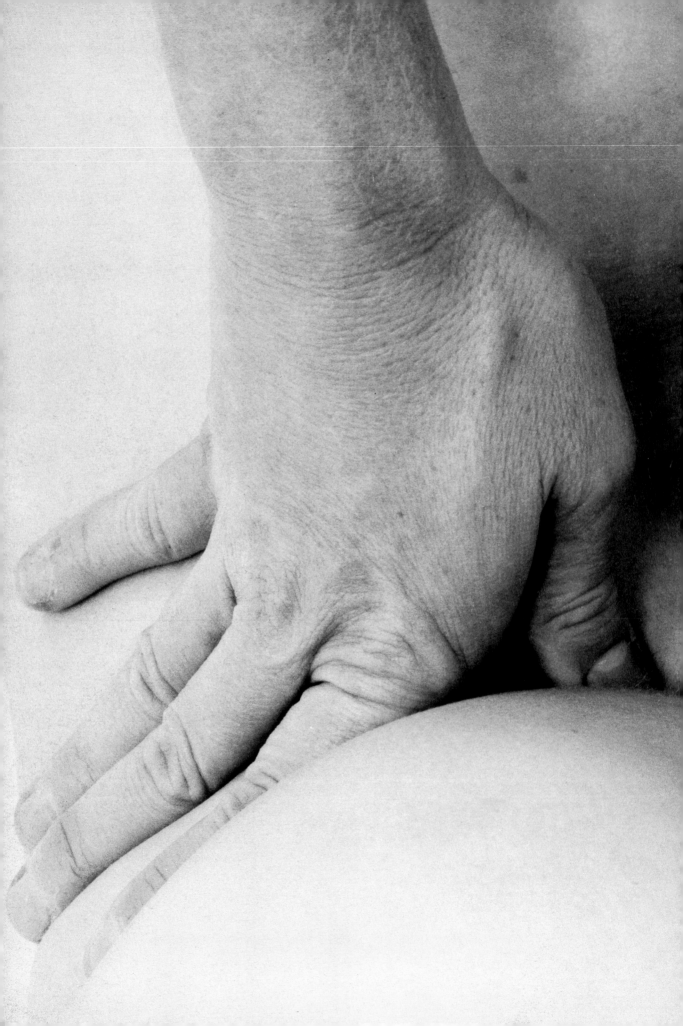

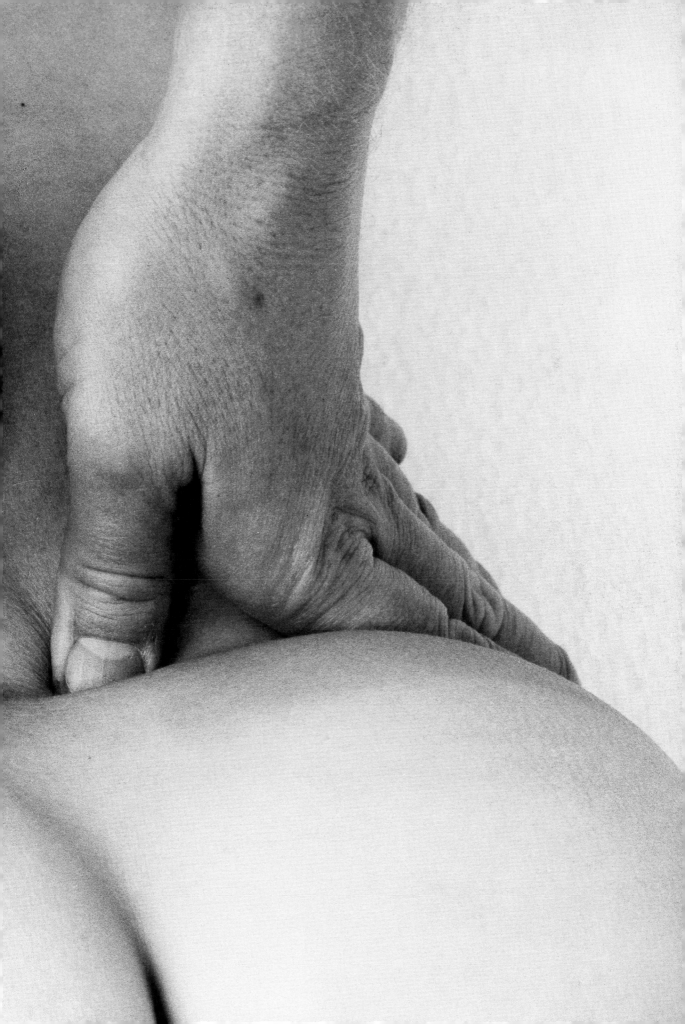

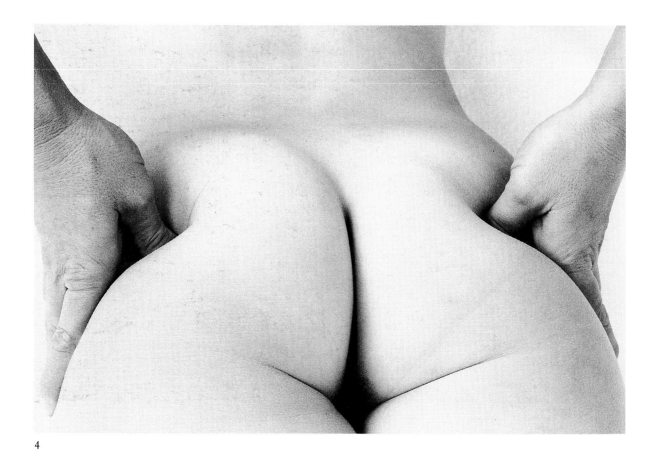

4

4. Working the gall bladder points

This technique is intended to relax the pelvic muscles and to relieve any pain in the sciatic nerve.

Use both thumbs to stimulate the gall bladder points, which are just to the outside of the centre of each buttock. Trust your intuition and, chances are, you will be on the right point.

5. Opposition stretch from pelvis to thigh

This movement helps to release the hip joint and pelvis. It will make your partner aware of the connection between the thigh and pelvis when the body moves in a diagonal stretch.

Kneel at your partner's right side, just below the pelvis. Place the heel of your hand on the nearest edge of the sacrum, and your left hand on the back of the left thigh. Perform stretching and rocking movements with your hands working in opposition to one another. It takes a little practice to get it right. Try to feel the stretch. Imagine your hands becoming one with your partner's body, so that you are perfectly connected and grounded. Without changing your position, work the other side.

This technique is the same as the opposition stretch described in the Fundamental Energy section (see the illustration on p. 25). As well as being important in the process of teaching people the principles of massage, it is a good technique for this stage of the pelvis massage.

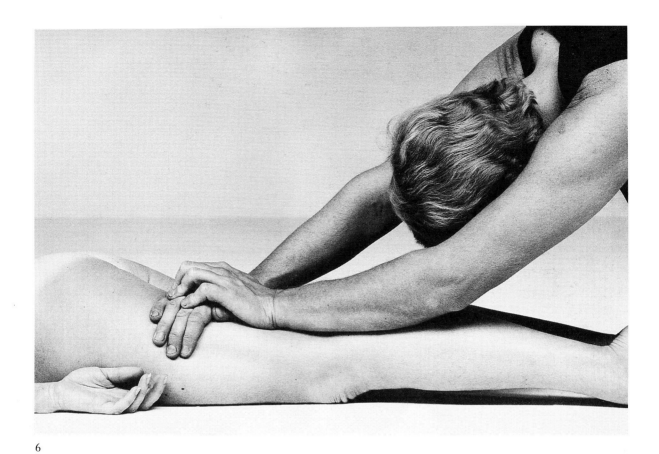

6

6. Back of thigh strokes

This is one of the best massage techniques for stretching tight, glued hamstrings which can cause tilting of the pelvis and aching knees. Repetitive exercise, such as weight training or running, can cause these muscles to become over-tight.

To massage the three hamstring muscles, move down and kneel next to your partner's left side near the ankle. For the left leg, use your left hand for the outer and centre hamstrings and your right for the inside one. For deeper pressure, place one hand on top of the other.

Stroke with your hands, putting pressure into the heel of your hands, from just above the knee up to the thigh joint. Maintain an even pressure throughout the movement. Use your weight and relax your hands, keeping your fingers in contact with your partner's body. Do each hamstring several times, then work the right leg. This is a stretching stroke, so you should make each movement as long and continuous as you can.

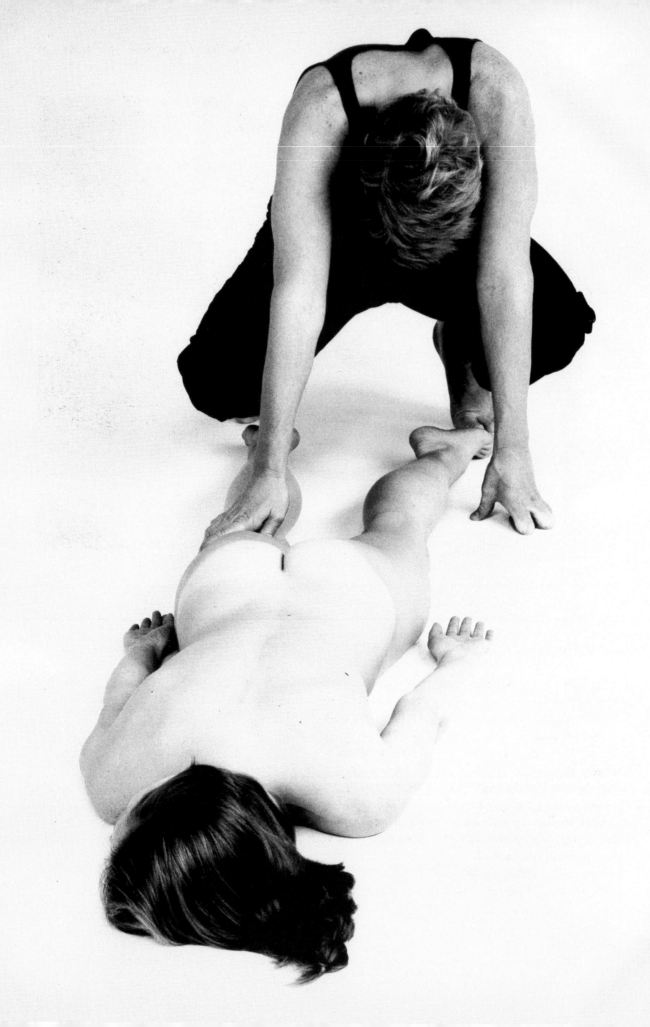

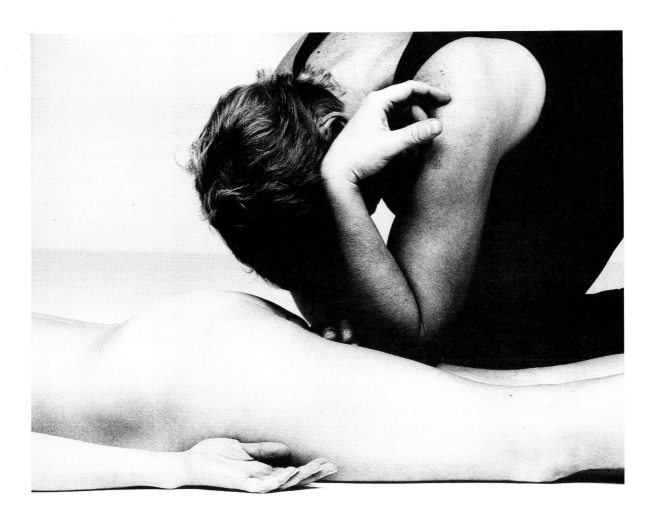

7b

7. Back of thigh points

This is a further technique designed to release tension in the muscles of the legs and pelvis. The bladder meridian travels down the centre of the thigh and the points are very deep here, so I often use an elbow or knee for more effect. Although you can exert a greater pressure with the knees and elbows, they are less sensitive than the fingertips so you have to take care. You need to be aware of your entire body in order to stay relaxed and generate energy which will be transmitted to your partner.

a) Stand by the feet and work the thigh, gently at first.

b) When you wish to increase the pressure, move closer to your partner and use your elbow.

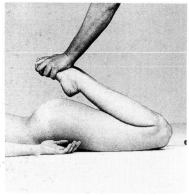

8

8. Leg to pelvis stretch

This simple technique lengthens
the muscles on the front of the
thigh. You should do it gently
and slowly as most people's legs
will not be as loose and flexible as
this dancer's.

Pick up the feet, one in each
hand, and stretch the lower legs
back to the pelvis. Hold for a few
seconds and release.

9. Opening up the joints of the lower body

This is a good technique for
releasing compression in all the
joints of the lower back, the hip,
the knee and the ankle.

Simply lift the legs by the
ankles so that the hips and pelvis
are slightly raised from the
ground, and the weight of your
partner's body will cause the
space around the joints to widen.

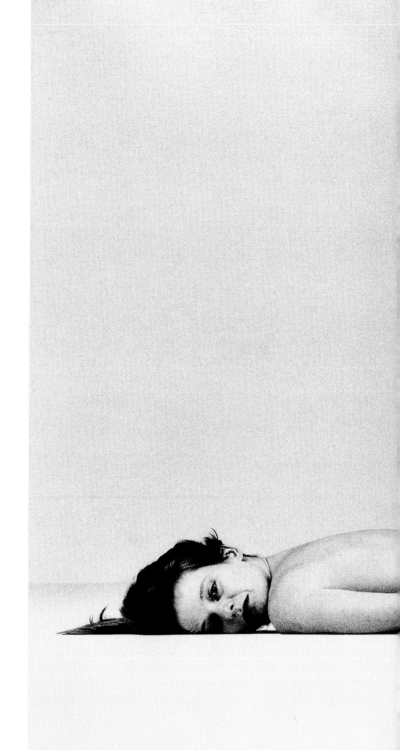

9

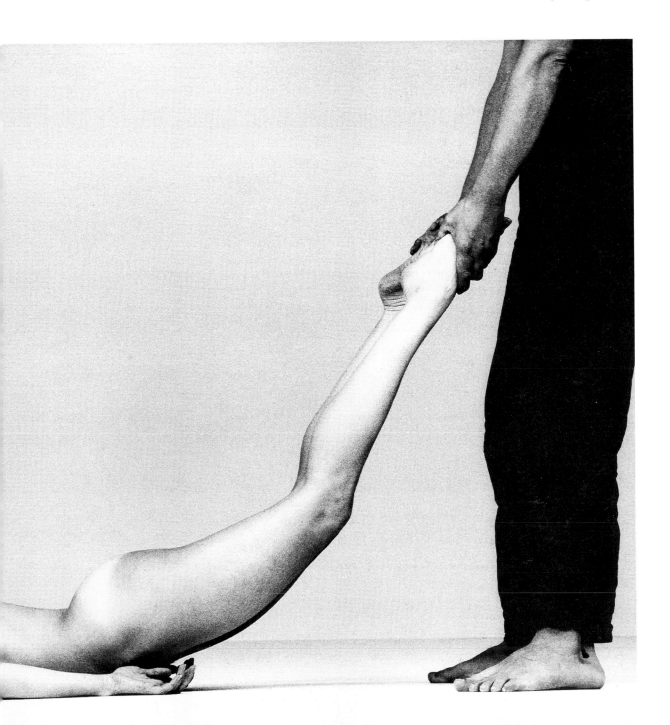

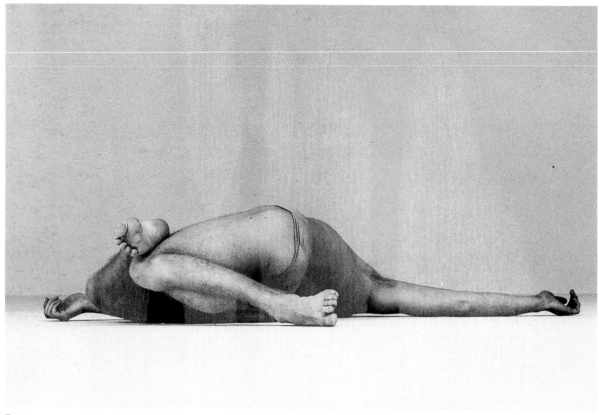

Ex 2a

CORRECTIVE RELAXATION EXERCISES

You and your partner can do these together or alone. The sequence helps to deepen the breathing at the lower centre and opens and releases the pelvis and thighs.

Exercise 1

This is an important exercise for stress and sexually related problems.

Lie on your back, with your knees bent and your feet flat on the floor, hip distance apart. Be sure that your legs are relaxed and balanced. Direct the breath deep into the abdomen; feel the breath lengthening the tailbone and pushing into the floor. Remember to pause at the completion of each exhalation, allowing all the breath to go out. When you have established a deep, relaxed rhythm, allow the legs to open out as you breathe in, letting your knees fall towards the floor. On the exhalation the legs are drawn together again. Keep your thighs relaxed; the movement is being generated by the breathing, not the muscles. Visualize the slow flow of breath being squeezed out between the legs. If you are relaxed, the thighs will begin to vibrate as you breathe out.

From the same starting position, roll up the spine, thus raising the pelvis a little, by pushing through the legs into the floor. Keep the movement confined to the pelvis and lower back as you are trying to open and create feeling in that area. The movement is done slowly, in time with the breathing. Roll up on the exhalation and down on the inhalation. After a few times, reverse the breathing pattern. The movement becomes a gentle rocking motion generated through the legs and the breathing.

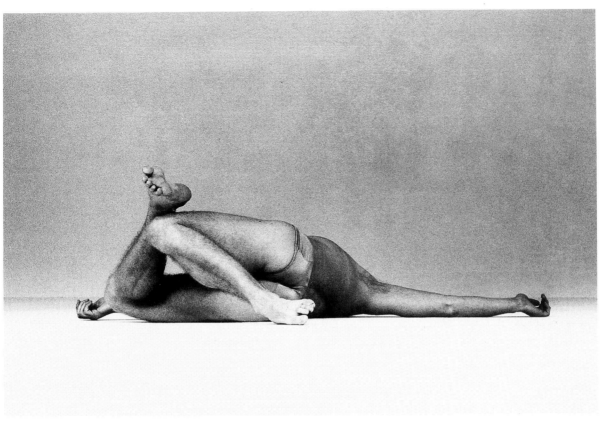

Ex 2b

Next try rolling in a circular pattern on the outer edge of the pelvis, still keeping your feet flat on the floor, hip distance apart. The gentle effort comes from the legs and is controlled by the breathing. Do the movement in both directions. The deeper you can bring the breath into the pelvis and the more relaxed you can be, the greater the feeling capacity will become. With all body movement it is important to use the minimum effort for the task.

Exercise 2

This exercise is designed to increase the flexibility and improve the positioning of the hip joint. It relaxes and co-ordinates the movement of the spine, giving fluid efficiency to the body.

Lie in the same position as for the last exercise, with your feet flat on the floor, hip distance apart, making sure that your legs are relaxed.

a) Place the right ankle over the left knee. Take deep, even breaths and as you breathe out allow the weight of the right leg to pull the left towards the floor.

b) As you breathe in, the legs will return to the starting position.

Feel how this passive stretch affects the hip joint and the whole of the spine. If you are completely relaxed, the head will be pulled the opposite way from the legs and your chin will be drawn towards the chest. Repeat the movement ten times, slowly, in time with your breathing. Then stretch your legs out, flat on the floor, and feel the difference at the hip joint.

Repeat the exercise with the opposite leg.

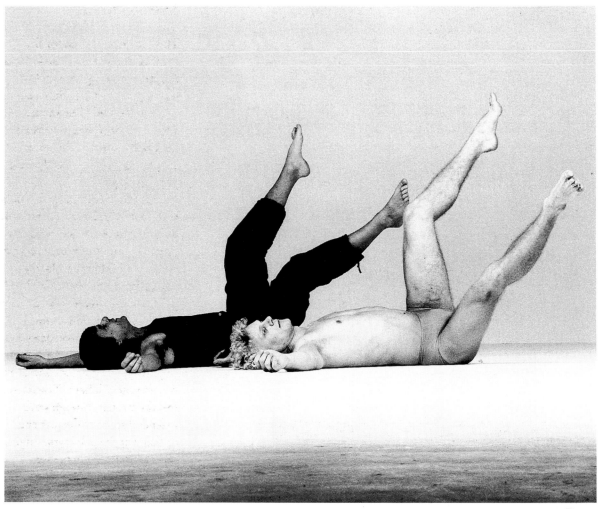

Ex 3a

Exercise 3

This exercise will teach you efficient body usage.

a) Lie flat on your back on the floor. Lift the feet high in the air. Bend the knees slightly and roll the legs right over to the right. Using the least effort possible, take the left leg up to the vertical again and over to the opposite side, and feel at what point the right leg naturally begins to lift. Allow the right leg to follow over to the left side.

Repeat this movement several times, rolling in opposite directions. Feel your shoulders lifting as you roll.

b) On the next sequence, use the arms and the legs. First, the right arm leads the movement and the right leg follows (c) before the left arm and left leg begin to rise. Take all your limbs over to the right. Then you can repeat the movement, starting with the left arm and left leg.

Feel the stretch across the spine as the body follows its most efficient route to complete the rolls.

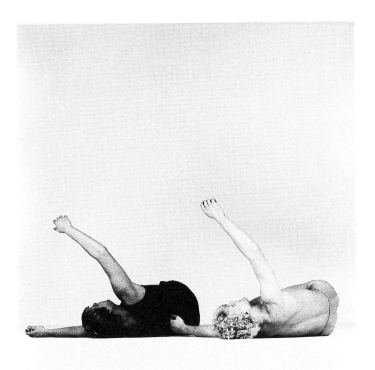

Ex 3b

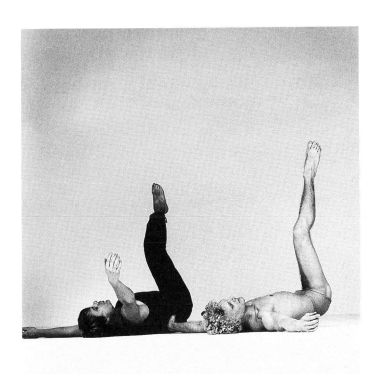

Ex 3c

Exercise 4

This is a good stretch for the spine. It teaches good body usage, the effort coming from below, leaving the shoulders open and relaxed. You will learn to trust in your relationship to the ground; the lower you can take your weight, the less you need to use your strength.

Face your partner, clasp hands and bend your knees, each of you pulling against the weight of the other. Be sure to lift the tailbone and extend the arms. The pull comes from right down in the pelvis, not from the shoulders and arms which should remain relaxed. The more you can bend your knees, lowering your centre of gravity, the greater control and power you will have. You need to feel the stretch through your extended spine as the power is initiated at the pelvis and thighs. (See the illustration on the following page.)

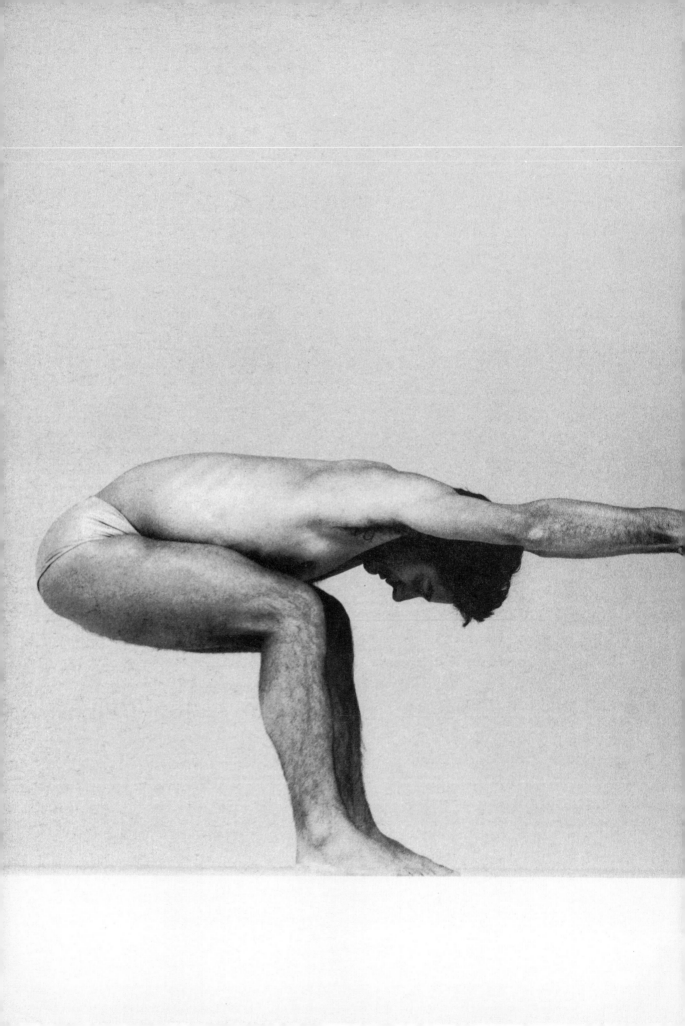

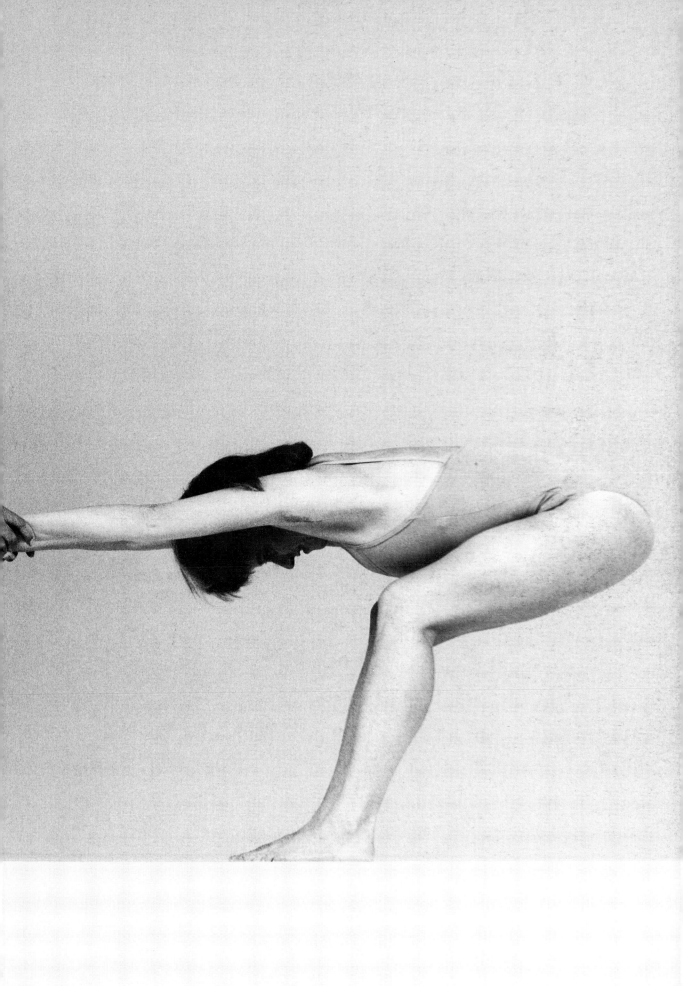

THE CALVES, FEET AND FRONT OF LEGS

Feet are our connection to the earth. They are constructed to be both strong, as a root support that must take the entire weight of the body, and sensitive. They are lined with nerve endings which, stimulated by contact with the ground, send healing energy to the organs and other parts of the body. To feel the earth's texture is to feel the texture of our own body. The lower we can take our centre of gravity, the greater our control and power. This is true for both our physical movement and our emotional well-being. The idea is to take our centre down to generate the energy to propel ourselves upwards and forwards. We need to direct our earth root as deep as we can, thereby increasing our capacity to handle emotion. The feet act as an outlet to dissipate emotional charge in the same way that an electrical current is earthed.

The importance of maintaining this physical sense of the legs and feet as ground is well demonstrated in skiing. You need to bend the knees, lowering the centre of gravity. You will have a relaxed feeling of control as you allow yourself to go with the downward pull. Leaning slightly forwards and lifting out of your heels, your body is able to make adjustments to changes of speed and movement. The moment you feel fear, however, the energy rises into the upper body and ceases to flow from your feet and legs so that you lose feeling and connection. The body goes rigid and you fall – hard.

To feel the legs and feet as ground helps us to live our experience in the body, to let go of fear. When we are overcome by emotional shock we lose this sense of body. We hold the emotional charge in our throat and chest and enslave our mind to endless chatter. The act of directing the unconscious tension downwards, as a physical energy, to the stillness of the centre and further down to the ground gives us an anchor, a source of personal and physical strength.

The base of the foot is composed of a tough web of connective tissue. Bound and secured by more than a hundred ligaments, 26 bones articulate at 33 places. These are shaped into a supporting structure composed of three arches: inner, outer and transverse. A healthy foot is sprung like a bow string. Power in the foot comes from its muscle connection to the lower leg. There are 12 muscles originating at the calf which aid stability and movement. They are all attached to the heel by the Achilles tendon.

Feet must be used to the full if they are to maintain their supportive strength. Habitual misuse and neglect, wearing restricting shoes and walking on hard, flat surfaces all prevent the muscles of the feet from working to their full potential. They become weak, flat and stiff, causing the structure above to sag, compressing the joints. The calves, especially at the ankle, reveal the truth about the way we use our feet. A healthy, functioning muscle is elastic to the touch. It works as a pump, moving fluids, nutrition and oxygen. It secures, supports and maintains space between the joints. A poorly used muscle, however, is swollen with waste and stagnant fluid, lumps of crystal form in the tissue, and it is painful to the touch. Feet need to be balanced, flexibly planted with fluid strength between the three arches.

Massaging the feet and calves brings attention to the area of the body that is often neglected. It stimulates and revitalizes feeling, and encourages movement of often congested fluids towards the distant heart. Stimulating the feet has a particular effect on the kidney and bladder meridians. They are associated with the element of water and also have a role in regulating fear, especially fear related to sexuality and change. The kidneys are related to the pelvis and jaw; if the feet and ankles are stiff, the pelvis and jaw will be too. Therefore, when working points of pain, especially at the ankle and heel bone, pay attention to the connection of the pelvis and hip bone and to changes of the jaw. An emotional release is common; it may be crying, perspiration or a change in the breathing pattern.

Fluid retention is common at the calf, making it swollen and painful to touch. People are often unaware of the condition of their calves until they are massaged. It is important to maintain muscular balance at the calf, allowing the foot to be planted centrally. You need to keep the muscles stretched, as short calf muscles will pull the entire body weight back onto the heels, compressing and swelling the ankle joint. If you keep the feet free of tensions they will be able to articulate as they are meant to.

After you have massaged the backs of the calves and feet, your partner will turn over. The main muscle group of the front of the thigh is the quadriceps. These four powerful muscles are involved in all leg movement and support the body against the pull of gravity. All four run the full length of the thigh attaching across the knee at the tibia. At the top, one of them attaches at the pelvis and the other three at the upper thigh.

MASSAGE TECHNIQUES

The following techniques concentrate on both the back and front of the calves, the feet and the front of the thighs. After working on the backs of the calves and feet, ask your partner to turn over to enable you to finish the feet and move up the front of the legs.

You are looking particularly for any areas of tautness or tension which you will be able to loosen by massaging. Some of the techniques and exercises will prove helpful in firming up weak muscles and weak joints and arches. Problems with digestion, menstruation, headaches, arthritis or a generalized lack of vitality are all related to emotional 'holding' and can be helped by stimulating the Shiatsu points in the leg. Pay attention to breathing patterns as you work. Emotional holding will mean that your partner's breathing is irregular. Watch out for any changes as these will give an indication of how they are reacting.

The front of the legs needs to be approached as a complete unit. Your aim is to create a sense of balance between both legs. The connection at the thigh joint should be flexible yet strong.

Reflexology is the method of working on the feet and ankles to diagnose and heal problems in the rest of the body. You can either incorporate it into the massage or make it a separate treatment. Massaging the feet exerts a beneficial effect in general on the body even without the use of specific reflexology points or with reference to just half a dozen points.

You can see from this photograph how differently people stand. The woman on the left is well balanced and lifted, her feet are well planted and her legs are identically shaped. The man on the right, however, is heavily weighted on his legs, particularly the right leg, and both heels roll in, thus weakening the ankles and tightening and unbalancing the calves

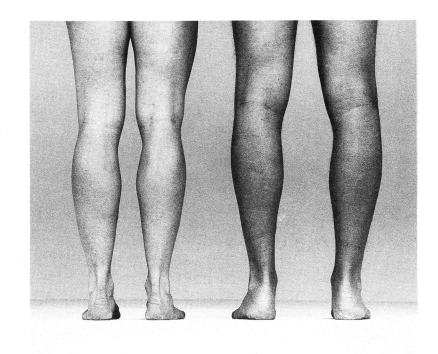

In this side view, the knees of the man on the right are hyperextended, pushing the weight back on his heels and shortening his calf muscles. By comparison, the woman has flexible, well-extended calf muscles

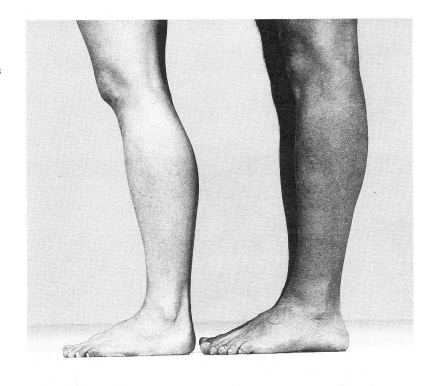

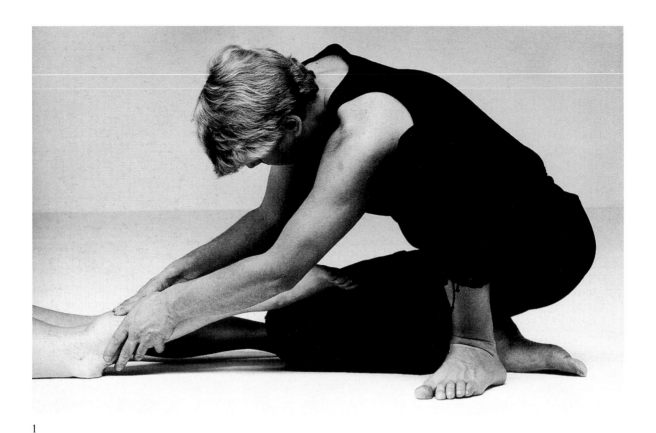

1

1. Calf strokes

With this technique you are aiming to move fluids up towards the heart, to restore the efficient circulation of the blood, thus improving the vitality of the muscles.

Your partner should be lying on their front, with you kneeling at the feet. Lift your partner's right foot and place it over your thigh. When doing massage and working points it is useful to support the foot in this way as it takes pressure off the ankle joint and gives a firm support to work against.

Start at the outside side of the calf at the ankle and, with your thumbs together and pointing up the leg, stroke a line straight towards the knee. Again from the ankle, but this time starting an inch nearer the Achilles tendon, repeat the stroke up towards the knee. Work your way to the inside of the calf, moving at one-inch intervals and applying long, deep strokes. Use equal pressure throughout the movement and be sure you keep to the line of the muscle. Repeat the movement on the left calf.

You should be able to sense the quality of the muscles as you work. Do they feel elastic or dense and compressed? Is there an imbalance in the strength of the muscles as you work from the outer edge inwards? If the leg is habitually turned outwards, the outer muscles will be over-used and tight, whilst the inner muscles will be weak, often allowing the foot to roll in, breaking down the inner arch.

2. Working the Shiatsu points in the calves

You are aiming to create feeling in the lower leg, to bring your partner's attention to the condition of their calves. The calves and ankles are associated with the emotions. You may find, amongst others, three bladder points, two in the centre of the calf and one just above the knee on the inside. There are also points at the ankle, the ankle bone and the heel. Do not worry so

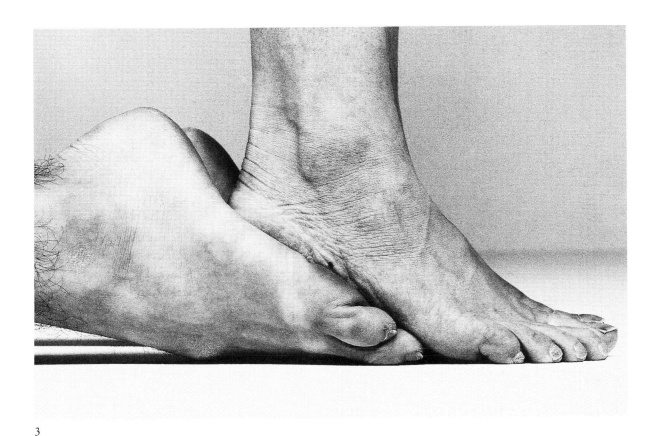

3

much about finding the specific points; it is more important to find painful points.

Remaining in the positions described for technique 1, use your thumbs and the tips of your fingers and work one calf at a time. Hold the points for 10 to 15 seconds, painful ones for longer. Then work on them both together, feeling the connection between the two and concentrating on balancing the energy. You need to work with a focused physicality, sensing the energy in your hands.

develop, right down in the feet, a sense of energy and of the correct use of the body's weight.

You can put a folded towel as support under your partner's feet. Stand facing away from your partner and place your heels on the under side of their feet. Relax, bend your knees slightly and balance your weight. Lean your weight back into the heels. Work the entire foot by subtly adjusting your weight and position.

3. Heel to heel

Use this technique to give a sense of grounding. It will help you to

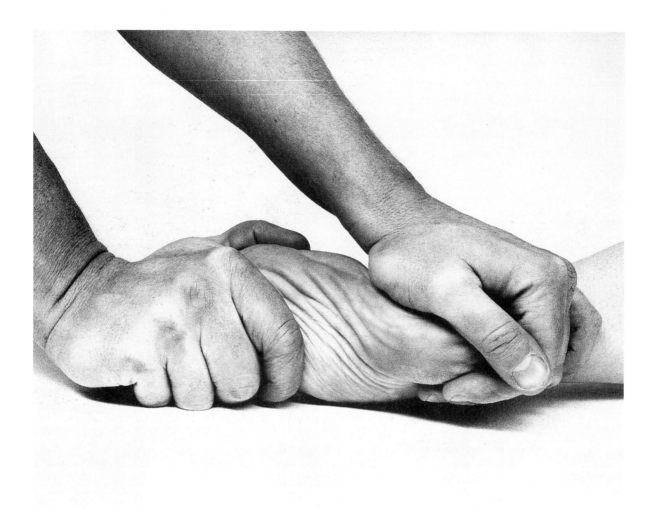

4a

4. Massage strokes for the feet

Feet tend to be stiff, lacking vitality and feeling. When you massage them you should stretch and twist them, opening and freeing movement in the joints (a). You can also stimulate the muscles and connective tissue with deep thumb strokes (b). You need to be active, using the energy of your whole body as you work with both hands.

You can also at this stage work some of the reflex points, but I prefer to leave them to later (see pp. 81, 84-7).

When you have finished massaging the feet, ask your partner to turn over.

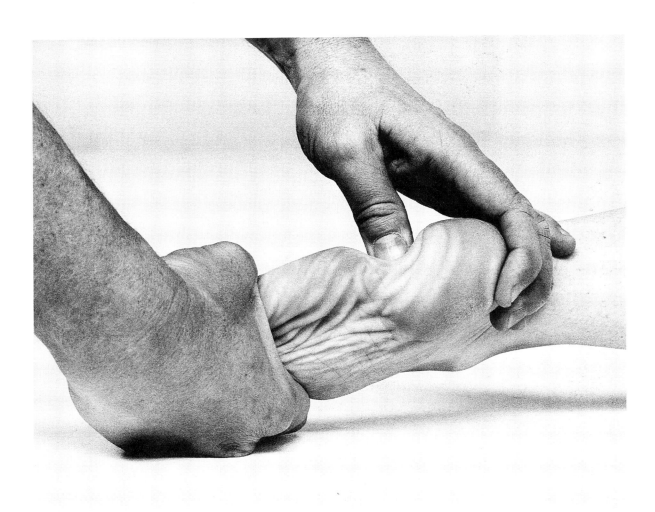

4b

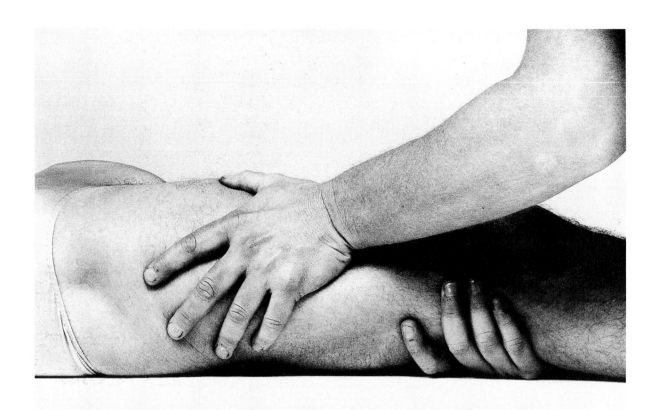

5a

5. Massaging the front of the legs

It is important to approach the front of the legs as a complete unit. Massage them using a sequence of continuous strokes, point work and stretches. The massage movements are interchangeable, but the treatment will be most effective if you alternate stretching and

massaging. You should interplay all the movements while maintaining a visual image of creating space in the joints, releasing muscles, stimulating points and balancing the relationship of the legs to the pelvis. Work slowly and remember to watch the breathing.

a) Lengthening the quadriceps
With your partner lying on their back, kneel next to their right leg. Massage with your entire hand for these thigh strokes and use your centre and body weight to direct the energy into the heel of the hand. Work the inner thigh with your right hand and the centre and outer muscles with your left. You need to work deeply and evenly along the entire

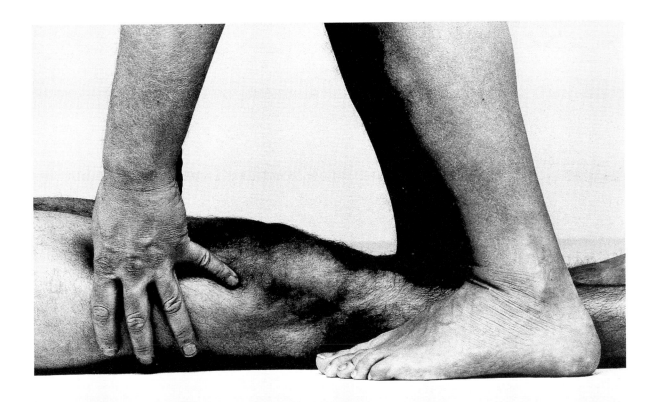

5b

length of the muscles from the knee to the thigh joint, keeping directly in line with the muscle.

Do several strokes on each muscle group, inner, centre and outer, then work the left leg. Dancers and athletes can often be very tight in the quadriceps as a result of overworking these powerful muscles, so the treatment needs to be deep to stretch and release them effectively. This can be painful, so work carefully and watch the breath. Massage just below the level of pain.

b) Applying deep stimulus in the thigh Stimulate the points of tension with the thumbs or the heel of the hand. Do not worry about meridian lines on the thigh as they are very deep. Direct your energy and your power by leaning with your body's weight on the points of tension. The effect will stimulate energy deep in the tissue. Start the movement gradually as you breathe in and then gently lean your weight as you exhale. The thighs are often held tight as a result of repressed anger and sexual tension. This technique can result in a powerful emotional release.

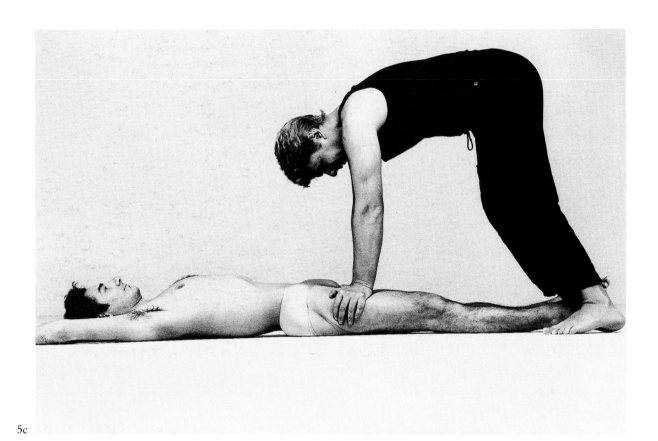

5c

c) Relaxing the thighs Move
your hands to the insides of your
partner's thighs. Use your weight
to stretch and open the pelvis-
thigh connection. Add a rocking
motion for greater effect.

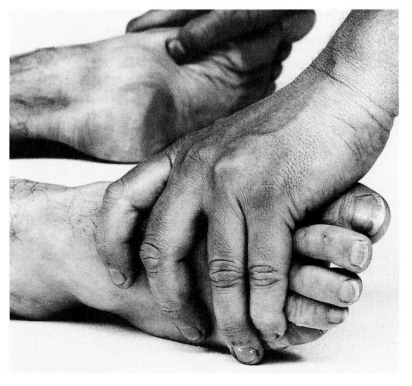

5d

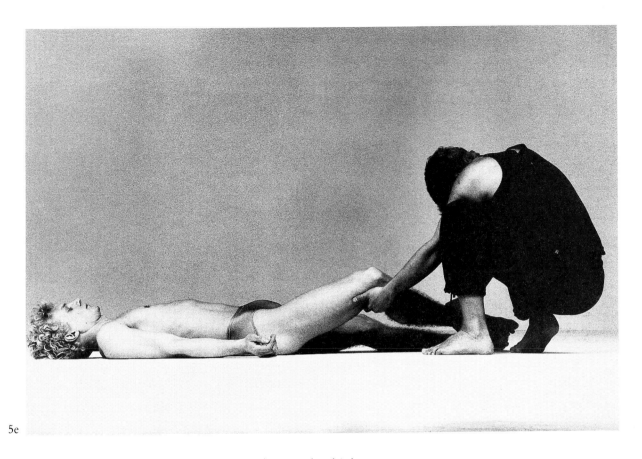

5e

d) Using points on the feet to relax the legs Standing or kneeling at your partner's feet, use both thumbs to stimulate the points at the inner heel bones and along the inner edge of the shin bones. Work both legs at the same time from the knees to the feet. The points can be sensitive so work carefully, breathing in as you approach the point and leaning your weight into the point as you breathe out.

Massaging the calves in this way is particularly important for releasing withheld anger, relieving stress-induced sexual problems, for resolving the problem of fluid retention and for alleviating muscular cramp.

e) Releasing the thigh joints Place your left hand under the right knee and your right hand at the ankle. Lift the leg, turning it outwards and gently pull and release a few times. This will free tightly held thigh joints. Work the left leg in the same way.

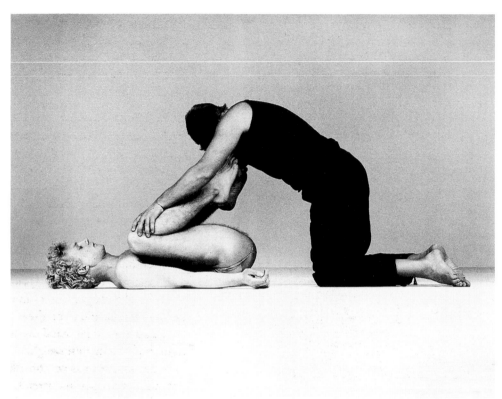

5f

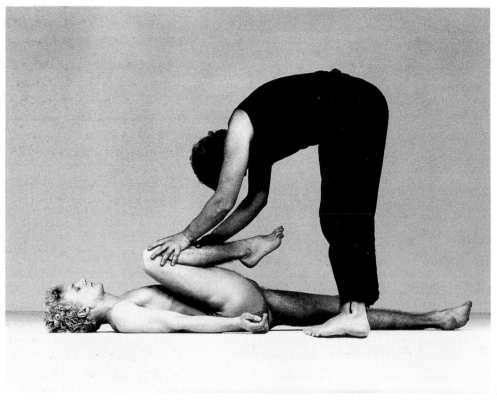

5g

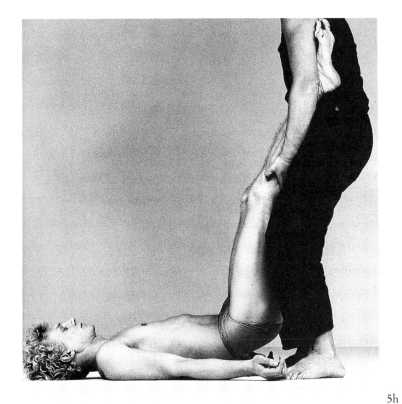

5h

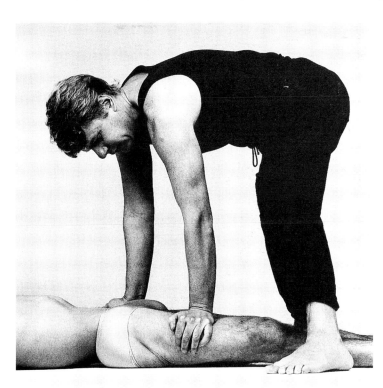

5i

f) Stretching the thighs   Take each leg in turn and lift it towards the chest in order to stretch the muscles of the thigh and release tightly held hip joints.

g) Stretching the lower back   Lift your partner's legs up together as you breathe in. Using the weight of your body, gently push both legs towards the chest as you breathe out in order to release the tautness in the lower back and thigh muscles.

h) Opening the pelvis   Standing over your partner this time, place your right hand at the top of the pelvis bone (the ilium) on their left side and your left hand on the right thigh. Lean your weight into the movement as you breathe out in order to open and stretch the pelvis-thigh connection. Add a gentle rocking motion if you wish to increase the stretch. Then work the opposite stretch.

i) Releasing tension in the joints   Lift the legs from beneath the knees in order to release and open out the space between the joints at the lower back and thighs. Hold the position for 10 to 15 seconds.

6. Working the reflex points on the feet

When you have finished the front of the legs, you can work the foot points. This is a convenient stage to do a little reflexology: your partner's legs and feet are warm, and your partner is lying face up – the best position for this treatment. (See pp. 84-7 for information and techniques.)

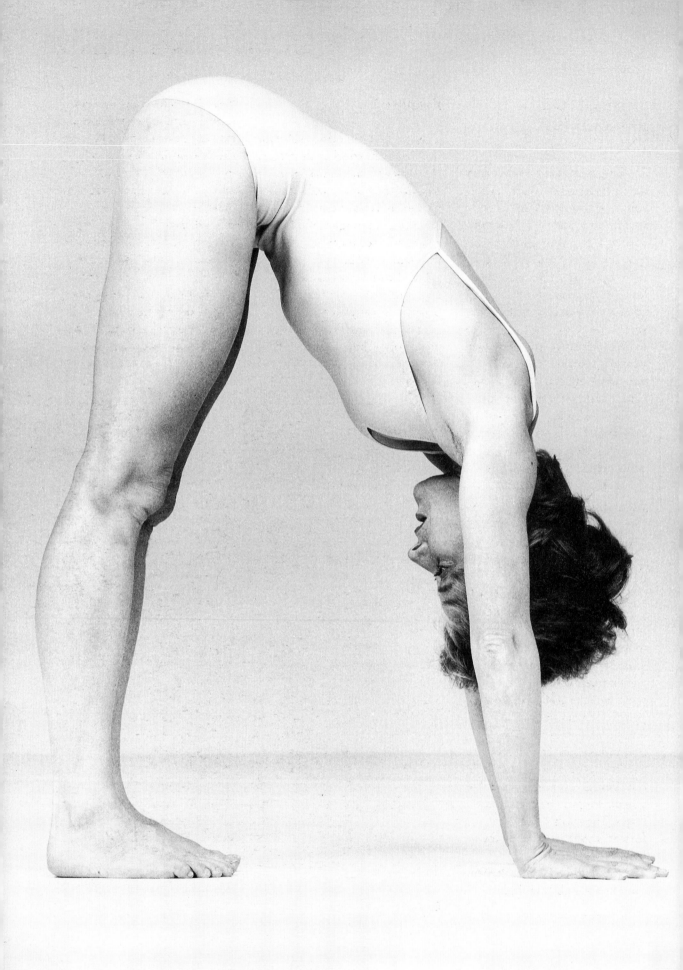

CORRECTIVE RELAXATION EXERCISES

The best exercise for the feet is to use them correctly. Walk in the countryside on grass, barefoot or in soft shoes, and sense how you need to soften yourself to the ground, how your knees have to relax and your centre of gravity lower in order to absorb the impact of the uneven surface of stones and earth. The feet need to work in a positive, strengthening way to oppose the negative, weakening effect of tight shoes on hard, paved surfaces. When the feet are weak and poorly used, the calves will also be weak. Simple exercise introducing small adjustments to the posture can create significant changes.

Exercise 1

This is a good exercise for stretching and balancing tight calf muscles.

Stand upright with your feet parallel and take your weight forward, bending at the waist as if to touch your toes. Keep your knees straight. Then take your weight further forward so that you touch the ground in front of you. Walk your hands further out, keeping your heels on the floor. Make sure your feet remain parallel as you want to stretch the calves evenly. It is important that you do not push back into the knees. The knees should move forwards over and beyond the feet as you bend.

If this exercise is difficult, bend your knees slightly at first.

Exercise 2

This exercise will help to solve the problems caused when the feet are weak and unable to support weight. The heels roll in and movement is transferred onto the outer toes, causing painful calves and misaligned posture throughout the body.

Stand with your feel parallel and your weight centred and balanced equally on both legs. Be sure your knees are relaxed; not locked or pushing back into the heels. Rise slowly up onto your toes, lifting through the body, extending the spine and keeping the head upright, then slowly lower your weight again. Do the movement slowly and evenly so that the feet and calves are strengthened. Come up as high as you can and hold the position for 10 to 15 seconds. You need to 'pull up' and feel the strength of the inner thigh muscles in order to hold the position. Be sure that you are pushing up onto the big toe and your feet are parallel.

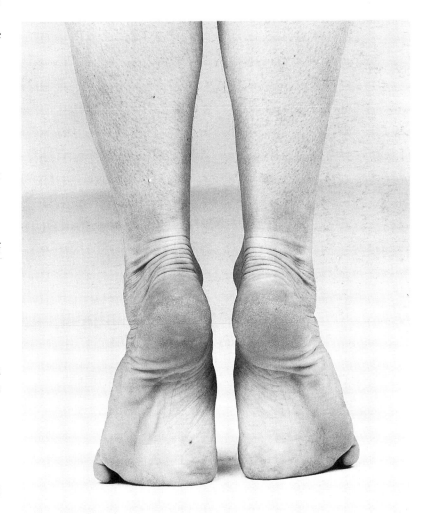

Ex 2

Ex 1

Exercise 3

As we age, our feet and legs weaken. This exercise will help to keep them strong.

a) Lie on your back with your feet flat on the floor and your knees bent. Lift your right leg so that your foot is raised above you. Push slowly through the foot, extending all the muscles. Relax and push again. This exercise is not merely a matter of flexing; you are trying to use all the muscles and joints to give them flexibility and strength. Do the same with your left foot.

b) Next make a circular pattern in a clockwise direction with the whole foot, stretching and working all the muscles and joints in the foot and ankle. Do 10 circular movements in each direction on each foot. It will be painful as it is hard work to find movement within stiff feet.

REFLEXOLOGY

Reflexology uses similar pressure points and concepts to those of acupuncture. It has, however, been developed as a separate system, first by an American called Dr William Fitzgerald in the early part of this century. His basic principles for 'zone therapy' – that the body can be divided into zones, and pain or disease in a certain zone relieved by applying pressure to corresponding zones on the hands or feet – were further developed by a compatriot therapist, Eunice Ingham. She worked with great enthusiasm to popularize reflexology, as it became, in the 1930s and until she died in 1974. (The International Institute of Reflexology was set up to continue her work.)

The idea is that the foot is an image of the entire upper trunk. If you place a picture of both feet on the back, one on either side of the spine, you will see how the big toe represents the head, and the place just before the hard surface of the inner heel represents the tailbone. The kidneys, being on both sides of the spine, have points on both feet, while the liver is reflected only on the right foot and the heart only on the left.

The feet are covered with nerve endings which direct energy to all the organs, glands and the whole physical structure. You can learn to diagnose problems in the rest of the body by analyzing the feet. Then, by working to create a free flow of energy in the feet, you can cause the corresponding organ or gland to heal. (The hands have similar reflex points but, because they are more frequently flexed and stretched, they need less treatment.)

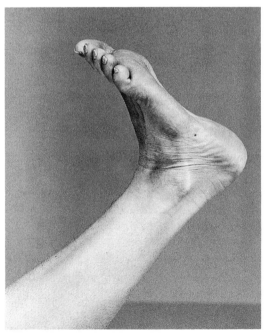

Ex 3a

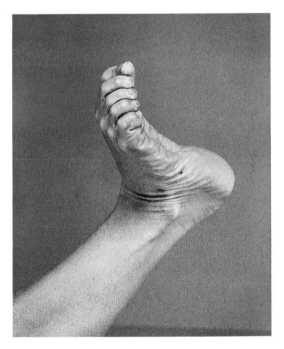

Ex 3b

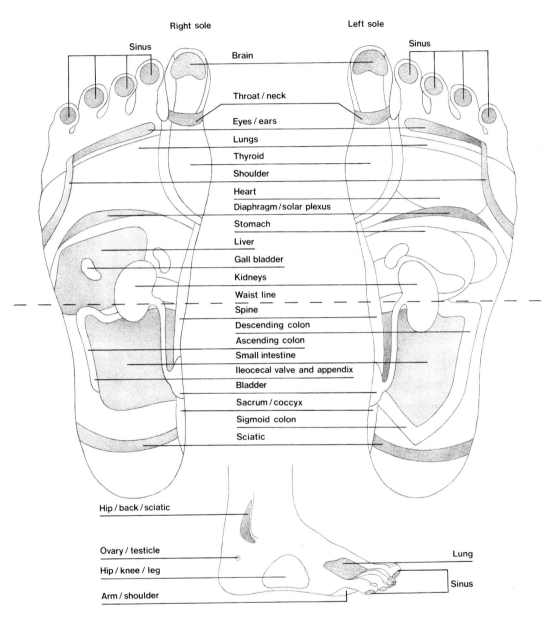

Right sole   Left sole

Sinus   Sinus

Brain

Throat / neck

Eyes / ears

Lungs

Thyroid

Shoulder

Heart

Diaphragm / solar plexus

Stomach

Liver

Gall bladder

Kidneys

Waist line

Spine

Descending colon

Ascending colon

Small intestine

Ileocecal valve and appendix

Bladder

Sacrum / coccyx

Sigmoid colon

Sciatic

Hip / back / sciatic

Ovary / testicle

Hip / knee / leg

Arm / shoulder

Lung

Sinus

Right outside

This diagram shows the reflexes, located on the soles of the feet, that refer to various parts of the body

Treatment

Your partner can either sit in a chair or lie on the floor on their back. For one session, 20 or 30 minutes is generally long enough. Beginners tend to spend too much time on a particular area or on a complete treatment because they tend to want to 'cure' everything in one go. If you work for too long, concentration may be lost, making it less effective, or the energy may even drain from your partner's body instead of flowing into it, thereby reversing the process. You need to know when to break the contact and stop. The healing process goes on long after the treatment has finished.

It is useful to use the chart on the previous page while you are working. Reflex points can be painful, and these may have a connection with the organ and joints specified in the chart. You must work just below your partner's level of pain tolerance as you need to find a balance between having them relaxed and yet attentive. It is no use working too softly, as concentration and effectiveness will both be lost.

Always work with both hands, using one hand to hold the foot whilst the other one works the points, so that one is the active stimulus and the other one is the ground. In order to focus your power, visualize the energy of your thumb going through the foot into your other hand. As always, the energy comes from an awareness of your own sense of grounding.

You should work the entire foot first and then concentrate specifically on the painful points. Work directly on one point for 15 to 20 seconds then move to

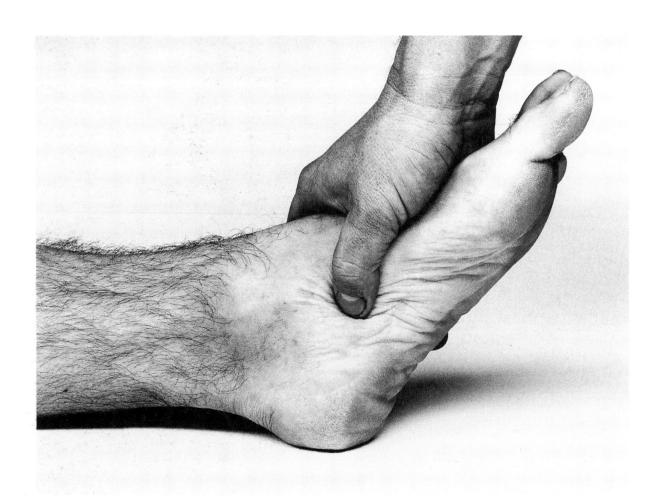

another area with the intention of coming back to stimulate the painful point again. Often it is good to give deep soothing strokes to relieve the intensity of directed thumb pressure.

Painful points are associated with blockages of energy; by stimulating a point you break down the congestion and allow energy to pass through. Be aware, and create a picture in your mind of the organ you hope to affect when massaging reflex points.

Following page: Healthy feet are strong, flexible and fully articulated

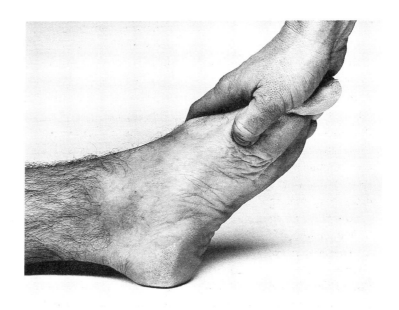

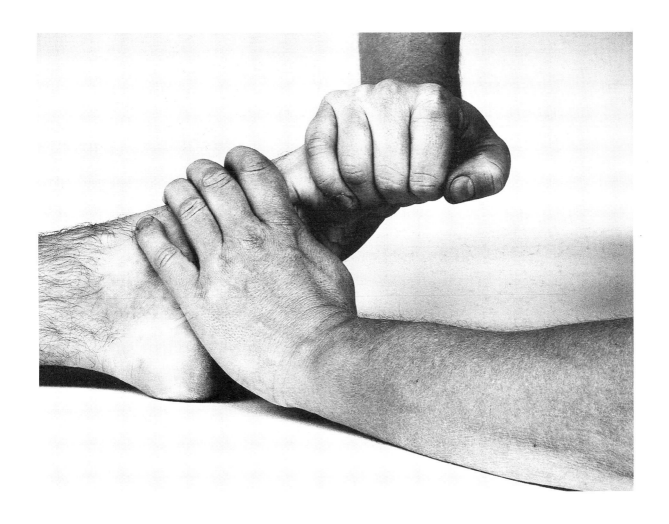

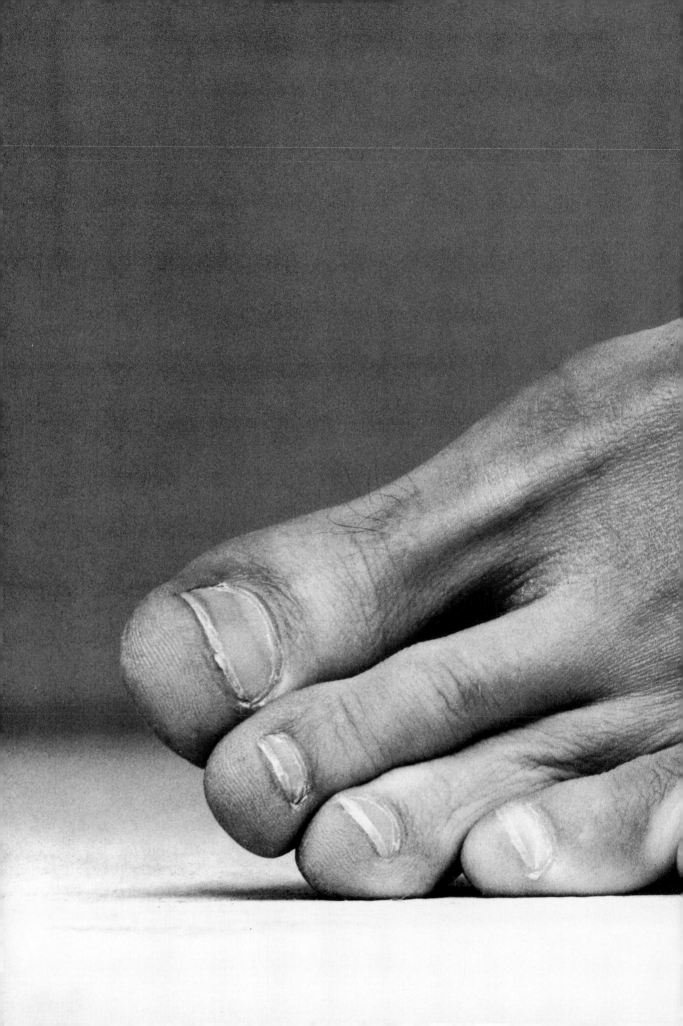

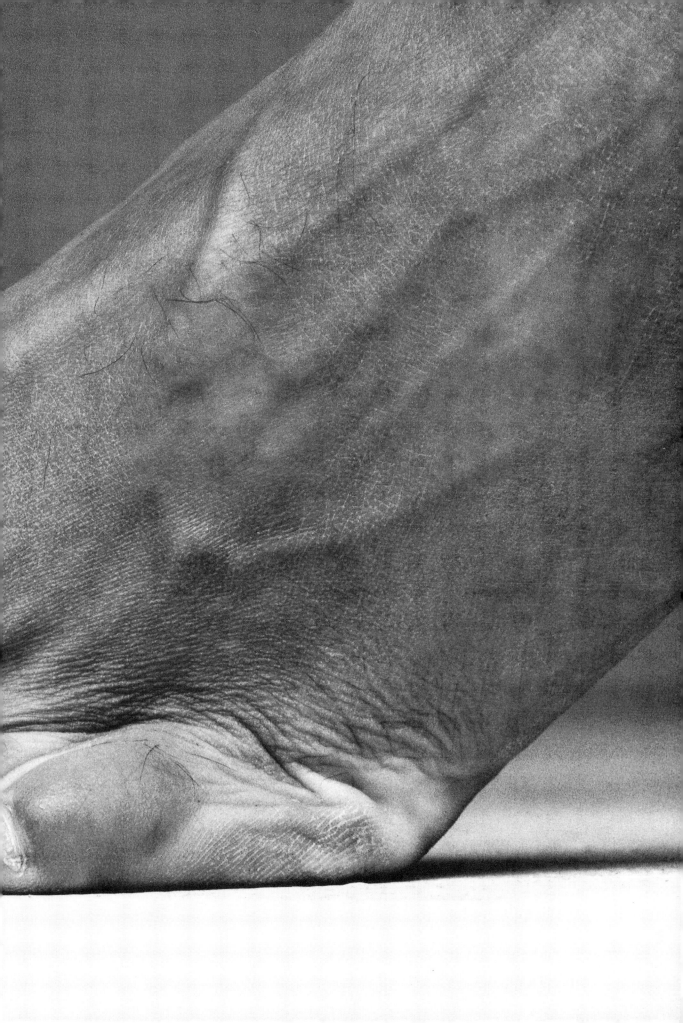

THE ABDOMEN AND CHEST

To massage the abdomen takes sensitivity. It is an important and personal area of the body. To the Japanese it is the hara, the centre of the body's strength, connecting spirit and ground, the 'divine neutral point' where energy is generated. It houses most of the body's vital organs of digestion and reproduction. Using Shiatsu, digestive complaints and other conditions related to the organs can be diagnosed and treated.

The abdomen is often a problem area, needing special attention. Dancers and athletes often over-develop the abdominal wall as they need to 'pull in' hard to get the power to jump. This often results in the organs being squeezed, preventing them from functioning properly. More often the abdominal wall is under-developed, allowing the organs to spill forward. We need to strengthen the deeper muscles along the spine, and ensure that the pelvis and hip joint are correctly positioned so that they can support the weight of the body. This leaves the outer layer of muscles free to fulfil their function of supporting the organs.

Breathing can be centred in the upper body or in the abdomen. It is essential to work with the breath to bring health to the abdomen. This will help you to feel the condition of the organs and to relax muscles that are over-developed or tight from emotional tension. We need to be physically strong at the abdomen, but it is also important to allow the breathing to relax and bring feeling to this sensitive area.

Corrective relaxation exercises for the abdomen are all concerned with deepening your breathing and increasing your awareness of your centre and the flow of energy; for this you will want to repeat the very important exercises from the Fundamental Energy lesson.

MASSAGE TECHNIQUES

It is important to pay attention to the breath. Some people get very tense at even the thought of having the abdomen touched and you may do better to avoid it. If you have any doubts, ask your partner. Rather than placing your hand directly on the abdomen, you could 'sneak up on it': first touch the sides, then slide round to the centre.

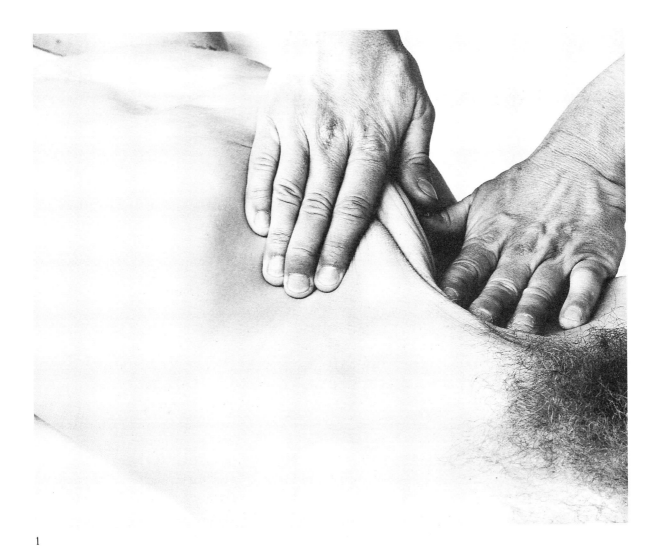

1

1. Massaging the abdomen

Using both hands, massage in a circular pattern. The strokes should go in a clockwise direction – the direction of digestion. Massage the entire outer edge of the abdomen, going under the ribs at the top and the pelvis at the bottom. Then gently squeeze and knead the central soft area of the abdomen.

Massage the entire abdomen gently at first, then work more deeply. Always stay aware of your partner's breathing pattern as it will tell you how the treatment is being received. If your partner's breathing becomes shallow, use a lighter pressure until they are relaxed.

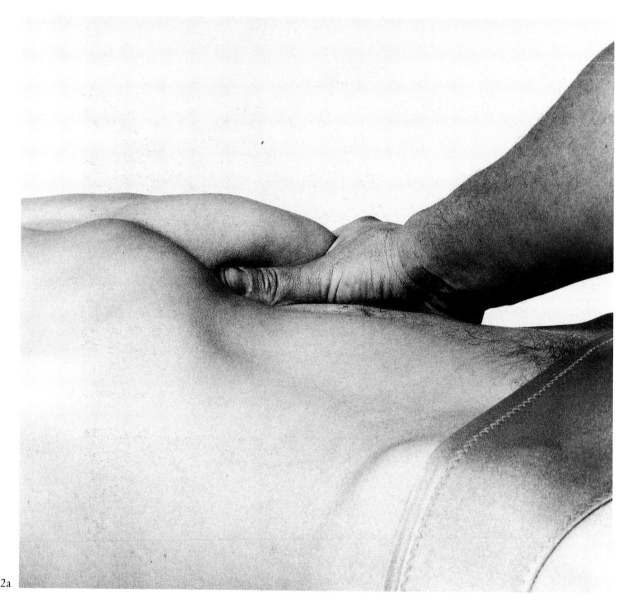

2a

2. Working the Shiatsu points

Working the points around the abdomen brings people's attention to the condition of the vital organs. The exercise is also designed to identify and relax tense, knotted areas. We often hold the muscles of the abdomen without realizing it.

a) Using the webbed space between the thumb and first finger, go gently under the rib-cage. The liver lies beneath the rib-cage to the right and the stomach to the left. If the area beneath the rib-cage feels tight, add a gentle rocking movement. If, on the other hand, you find that it is very loose, you can go deeper by using all four fingers,

held straight and flat, to work carefully under the ribs (b).

c) Work at the base of the abdomen as well, going in gently under the pelvic bones. Trace the intestinal tract in a clockwise direction, using your fingers softly and lightly.

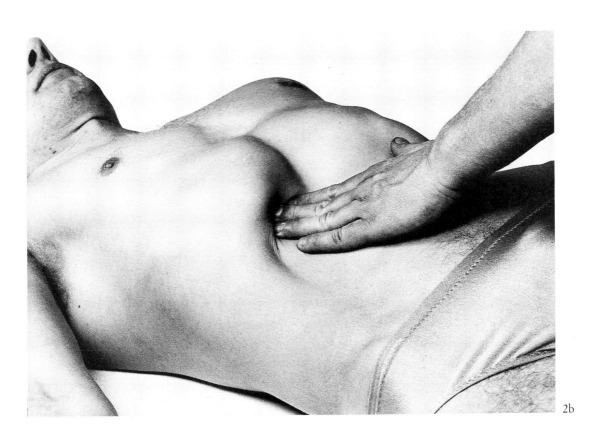

2b

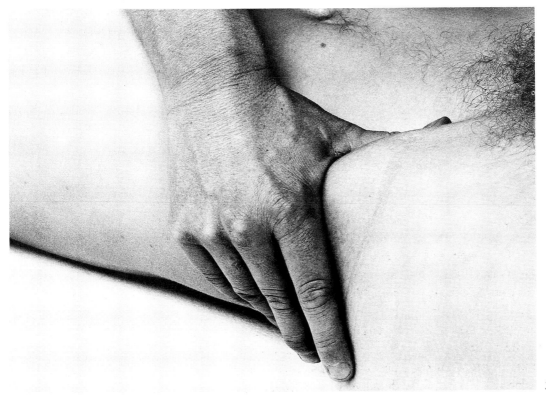

2c

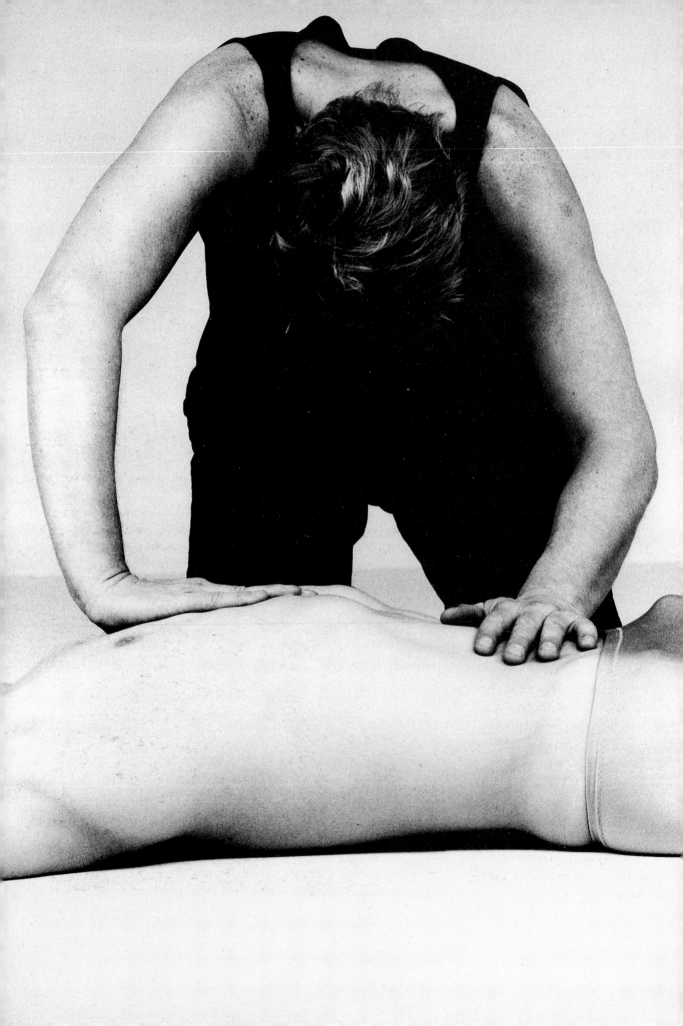

3. Passing energy

Working gently on the abdomen and chest can help to relieve digestive problems, emotional tension, colds and flu. You must stay relaxed so that you do not pick up other people's tensions and illnesses; if you try too hard to cure them, you're likely to end up with the same problems. Concentrate on staying centred in your own body and work with the image of passing energy, not of curing.

Place one hand at the centre of the abdomen and the other directly beneath it, under the lower back. Relax and focus on visualizing the energy as it passes between your hands, through your partner's abdomen.

4. Connecting with the chest and head

Several different positions are helpful for relaxing the energy centres of the abdomen, chest and head.

a) Place one hand on the chest and one on the abdomen to balance energy between the two centres, or try placing one hand just under the ribs and the fingertips of the other on the breastbone. Add a rocking movement for a calming effect.

b) Place your right hand across your partner's forehead and your left on the abdomen. You will probably be surprised by the different temperatures of the two areas.

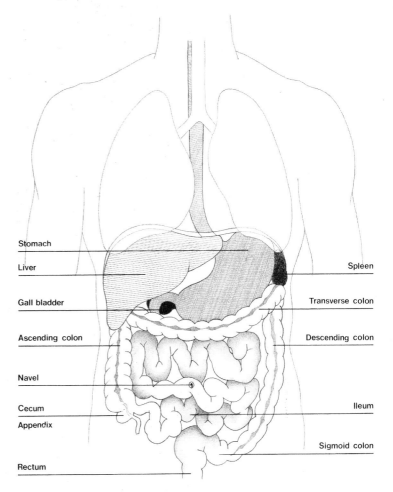

This diagram shows the abdominal area. It is important to have a good, upright posture so that none of the abdominal or pelvic organs are spilled out, squeezed or compressed.

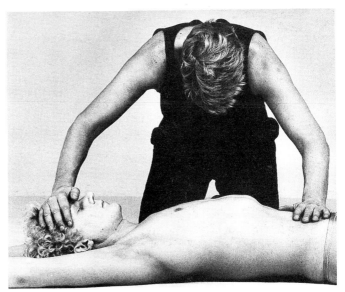

4b

THE SHOULDERS, ARMS AND HANDS

The shoulder girdle has a fragile relationship with the laws of gravity. It is superimposed on the rib-cage with only one bony attachment to the sternum at the front and a complex system of muscular attachments to the upper spine and head at the back. Whereas the pelvic girdle (with which a balanced relationship is essential for movement co-ordination) sits centrally and securely, the shoulder girdle is placed high above the centre of gravity. It is light and supports no weight which, combined with its primarily muscular attachments to the main structure, gives it great potential for freedom of movement, while leaving it vulnerable.

In order to maintain this ease of movement, the interwoven complex of muscles needs to balance. The rhomboids, teres, and trapezius are the main stabilizing muscles of the shoulder blade. Round shoulders indicate that the rhomboids have deteriorated. The common 'wing' look, when the scapulae stick out from the back, usually means the rhomboids and teres have developed unevenly, often as a result of bodybuilding. The trapezius muscles, which join the scapulae to the spine from mid-back to the head, are often bound and glued, causing high and tight shoulders.

The shoulders have become associated with physical work and masculine strength. It is fashionable to over-develop the chest, arms and shoulders, causing the centre of gravity to lift and the muscles of the upper back and shoulders to bind, which adversely affects posture and movement co-ordination. Ask someone to walk quickly or run and watch if the arms swing out to the side; if they do, the shoulders are tight. Musicians and people in occupations that keep them sitting for long periods often have difficulty with tension at the shoulders. This is a result of overworking the upper body instead of generating the energy and power further down. The tension builds up because the body, which is naturally active, is prevented from being so.

We rely on our arms as our physical means of communication. We need to feel that the expression of the arms is being generated from the spine, improving co-ordination and the flow of energy.

MASSAGE TECHNIQUES

As with the feet, the arms can feel disconnected. Generally, the problems felt in the arms such as numbness and lack of strength are caused by poor alignment of the shoulder girdle inhibiting the nerve and blood supply to the arm and hand. So adjustment of the shoulder is important for restoring co-ordination and releasing muscle tension, freeing the arms for expression. Massaging the hands gives them a feeling of connection with the body.

We have already worked many of the shoulder muscles during the lesson on the back, so in this chapter I will concentrate more on the arms and hands. It is probably easiest to do all the exercises for one arm and hand before moving over to your partner's other side to repeat them.

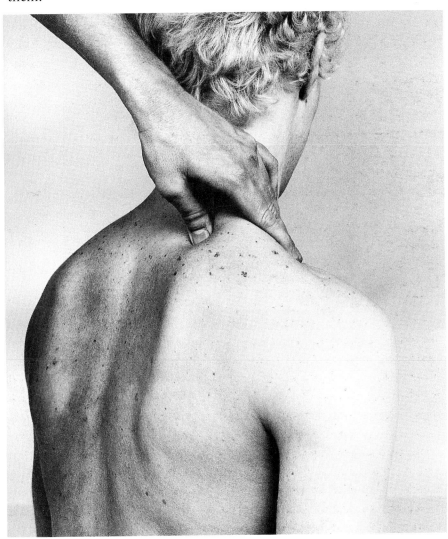

Adjustment of the shoulder is important for releasing tension

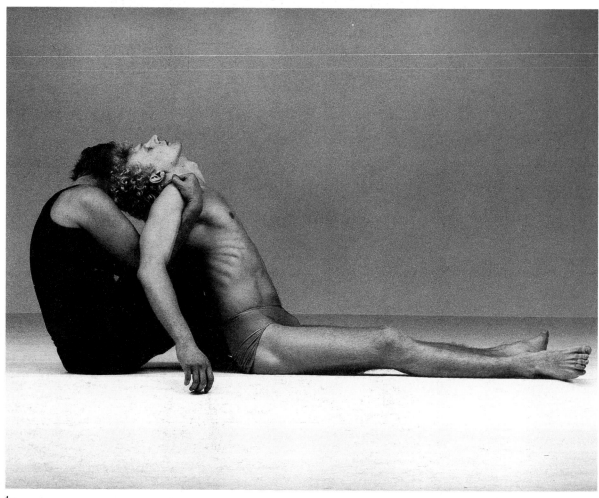

1a

1. Shoulder stretches

This is a wonderful pair of stretches for opening the chest and throat and releasing a tense, rounded upper back and shoulders. It will improve the breathing capacity.

a) Sit behind your partner and place your arms under and around the shoulders and your knees next to the spine at a point between the shoulder blades. Synchronize your breathing and, on the exhalation, pull your partner's back gently against your knees and stretch. Make sure that your partner allows their head to fall back against you. Do the movement several times, moving your knees higher each time. For people whose muscles are very tight this stretch may be uncomfortable. If it is – do not do it.

b) For the next stage of this technique, stand behind your partner and, taking hold of them by their arms, lift their arms up over the head and back towards you. Stretch the arms upwards as you breathe out, gently pushing into the back with your knees at the same time.

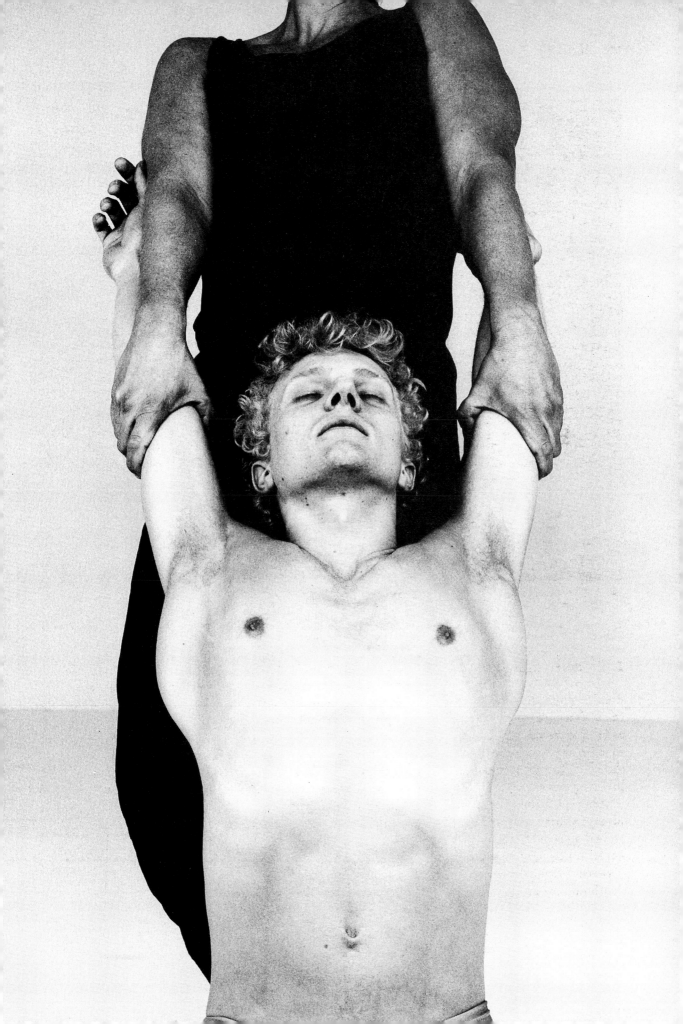

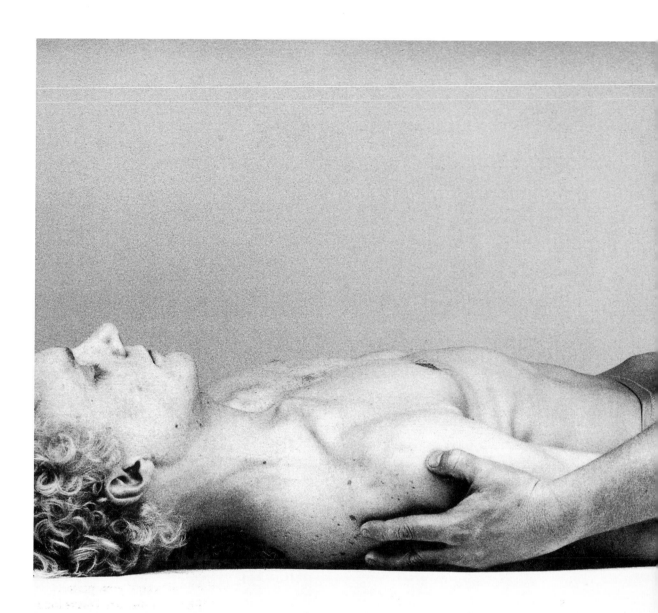

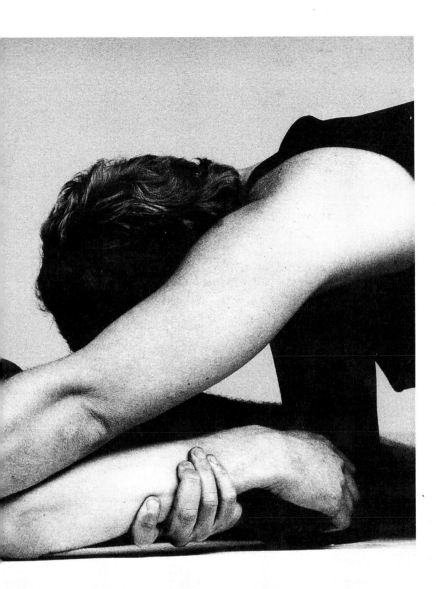

2. Adjusting the shoulders

This movement will realign the shoulders, improving the nerve connection and blood supply to the arms.

Kneel on the right side of your partner who is lying face up with their arms lying loosely out from their sides. Place your left hand under the shoulder and hold the forearm with your right hand. Pull the arm and shoulder towards you to widen and loosen the shoulder blade. Extend the movement out in different ways. You are trying to give your partner a feeling of separation between the arm, shoulder blade and spine.

Work the left arm from the left side.

3. Massaging the upper arms

This technique should restore feeling to the arms and relax tense muscles.

Kneel beside your partner, as in the technique above, but support the arm just above the elbow with the hand nearest your partner. With your other hand make long strokes from just above the elbow to the shoulder. The pressure should come from your thumb as you take the arm between your thumb and fingers. Be sure to cover the entire area. On the underside of the arm, take the movement up and under the shoulder to give a feeling of connection between the shoulder and the arm.

Work the other arm in the same way.

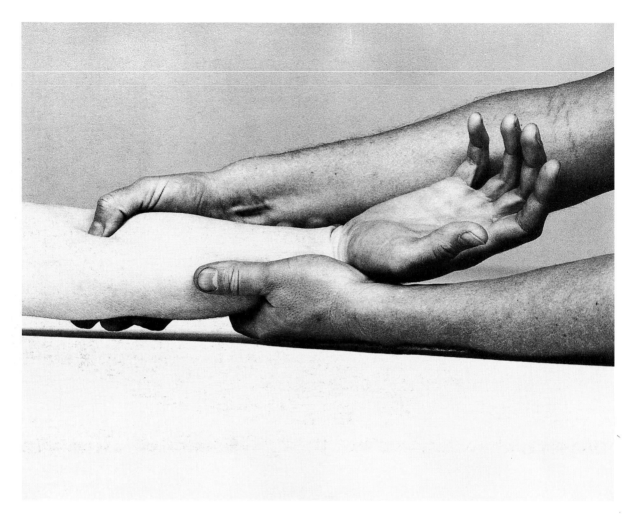

4. Massaging the forearms

Support the forearm just above
the wrist with one hand. Again
make long strokes, taking the arm
between your thumb and fingers.
You can also use direct pressure
with the thumbs to stimulate the
Shiatsu points related to
digestion, circulation and general
health.

5. Massaging the hands

Massage the hands as you do the
feet.

a) Use both hands to focus
your energy.

b, c and d) With your fingers
generally stretch and work all the
muscles and joints of the hand,
using the thumbs to apply direct
pressure to the Shiatsu points and
points of tension.

e) Extend and individually
massage each finger.

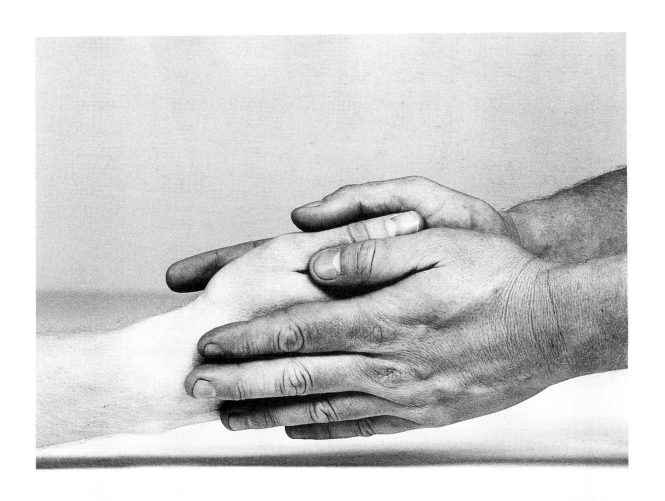

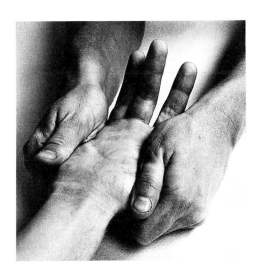

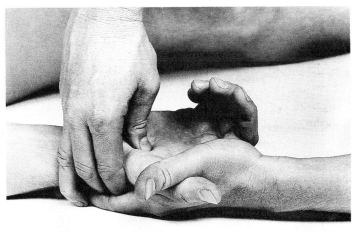

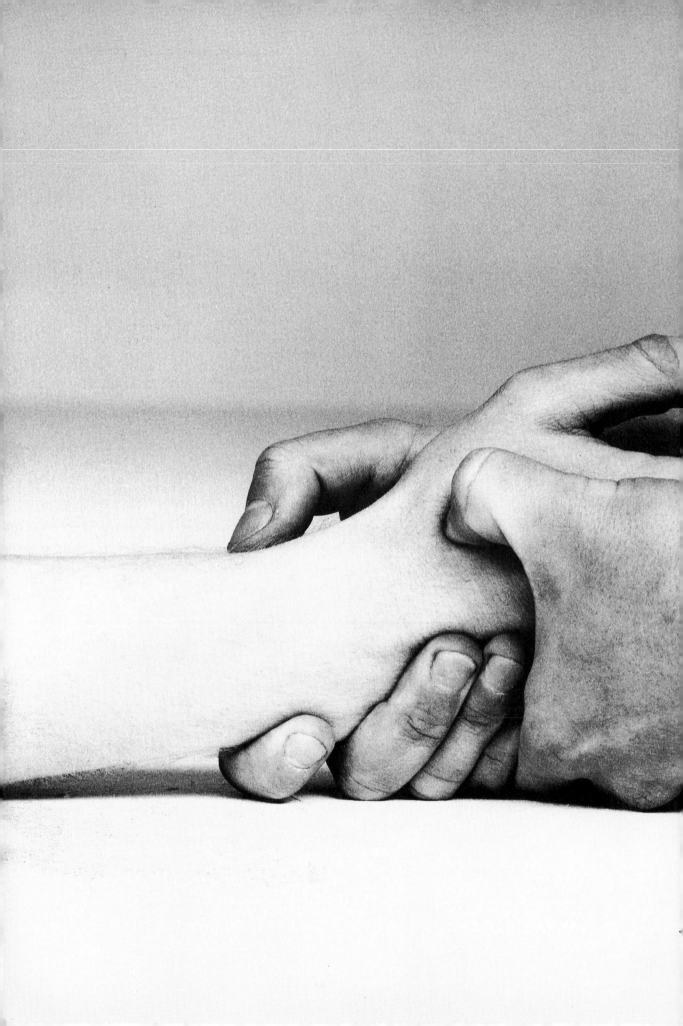

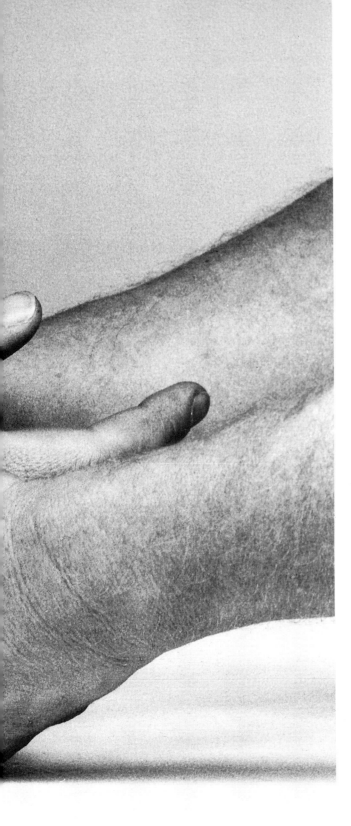

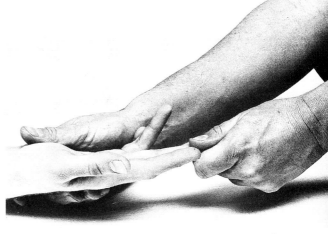

5e

5d

THE HEAD, NECK AND FACE

The skull is made up of at least 20 bones which are tightly interlocked with each other, an intricate pattern of nerves, blood vessels and muscles and just one joint – the jaw. The spinal cord continues upwards from the back inside the seven vertebrae of the neck (the cervical vertebrae) and into the skull as the brain stem. The neck forms a narrow bridge between the head (normally weighing between 12 and 15 pounds) and the trunk.

In a healthy, well-integrated body the head sits lightly and moves with freedom on the physical structure, allowing the face an expression of clarity, vitality and openness. A healthy person has positive perception and judgement and is intuitive, possessing a natural animal instinct to sense danger and change. Children are naturally like this. They radiate an alive sense of presence that is relaxed, fluid and alert to change. They have a natural quality of ground and centre, generating energy upwards through a lengthened spine and well-positioned neck.

Unfortunately, life without spirit or direction, an absence of grounding or earth connection, stress and bad postural habits cause the weight of the head to fall forward, and the image and physicality change. The connection between the head and the body is a vulnerable balance: although a deep web of muscle ties the skull to the trunk at the occipital junction at the second cervical vertebra, the weight of the head pulls naturally forwards. In a vital and active person this natural pull forwards is lifted with energy and gives focus and direction to the body's movement, as can be seen in the alert movement of animals. When a person is over-stressed and inactive, the weight of the head becomes a burden, putting strain on the superficial muscles of the neck, for example the sternocleidomastoid, and the trapezius. The muscles' main function of directing the freely moving head and shoulders is lost. The muscles shorten as the shoulders pull up and round, the head hangs forwards, cutting off the supply of blood, nutrition and energy to the brain and causing headaches, eye strain and a general lack of spirit. The expression of the face will reflect this stress and lifelessness.

The face gives an outward expression to our inner being, to the clarity of our mental activity and emotions. We have little control over the way our outer appearance maps an impression of our inner energy. It can reveal insecurity in the nerve reflex of rapidly blinking eyes or maintain dominance with an empty, hard stare. It can shape a blank mask to hide our fear or hold a fixed and angry look to keep people at a distance. Each of these expressions reveals more than we realize about our inner state.

In Chinese medicine the face's most important association is with the heart, but it is also used to diagnose the condition of all the body's organs. The shape of the head and jaw are related to the kidneys. Repressed anger, indicated by a tight jaw, will also mean that the pelvis and ankles are tight. The eyes, called the 'windows of the soul' (just as the pelvis is called the 'seat of the soul'), are associated with the liver. Vertical lines above the nose reflect the condition of this organ as well. The mouth and throat express the health of the lungs. The cheeks are related to the circulation of the blood. A healthy face should be moist and lively rather than dried out and drawn.

MASSAGE TECHNIQUES

The face is a sensitive and personal part to massage. You need to be relaxed and focused. Your partner will be very sensitive to what you impart. If your hands are stiff or nervous, or if you lose concentration and drift off, they will feel it at once. You need to feel the energy coming from your centre and not just from your hands. You will be aiming to relax and strengthen the many muscles of the face which are frequently formed into a mask of tension or have weakened and lost tone from lack of expression. In this head-dominated society, stress often causes a build-up of dense heat which can be dissipated by the energy of someone else's hands.

Although many meridians begin and end at the face and head, the Shiatsu points here are used more frequently to relieve local tensions such as headaches and eye strain. They can be used to diagnose tension elsewhere in the body.

The stretches will enable you to release the muscles in the neck where extreme tension can build up. You should bear in mind the vulnerability of the neck and work carefully. One of the neck exercises is at the end of the chapter, and of the massage, because it requires your partner to sit up.

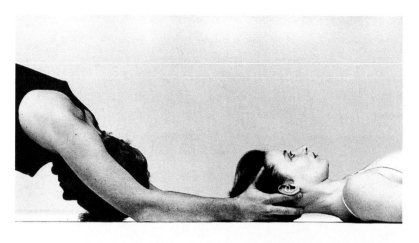

1a

1. Passing energy through the head

The first stage of this sequence assists deep relaxation and alleviates mental fatigue. The last stage will release the emotional tensions of the throat and is also effective for headaches. Energy will flow both ways throughout the movement and both you and your partner will feel calmer.

a) Kneel behind your partner – who is lying face up on the floor – well back from their head so that your arms and body are extended. Note that the forearms lie along the ground and the line extends through the rest of your body. This helps to relax and ground you so that energy can flow more freely. Place your hands, supported by the floor, under your partner's head. Relax and maintain this position for 30 to 60 seconds. This 'non-doing', finding the place of positive stillness within yourself, is often the hardest thing for the beginner to do.

b) From the same position, move your hands to opposite sides of the head. With your fingers directly opposite each other, imagine energy passing from one hand to the other, through your partner's head. Focus your attention – you should be positive, relaxed and receptive. You need to feel energy moving out from the stillness of your own centre. Make sure that your shoulders are relaxed so as not to cut off the flow of energy.

c) For the final stage of the movement, kneel or sit nearer to

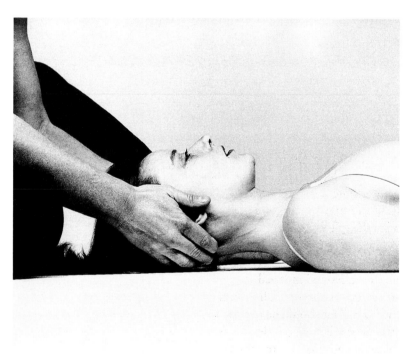

1b

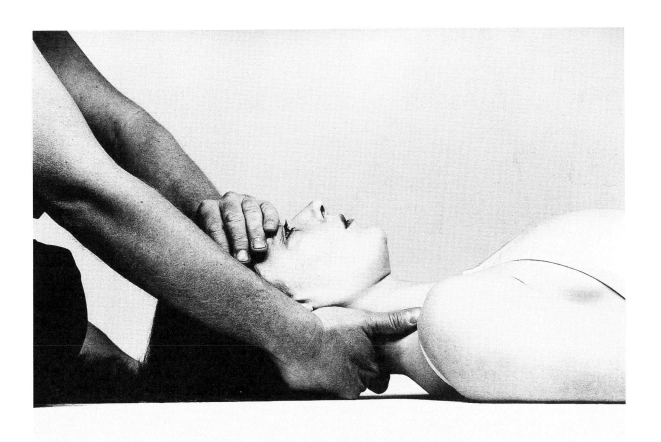

1c and 2

your partner's head and place one hand under the neck, the other on the forehead. (This is the starting position for the next technique.) Again you should hold a positive image in your mind of the energy passing between your hands. Be aware of your own and your partner's breathing. It should have become slower and calmer.

2. Extending the neck

This technique will release tight neck and shoulder muscles and align the spine.

Place one hand under the base of the skull and the other on the forehead. Extend the head straight towards you, in line with the floor. This should be a relaxed stretch; it is better to do less with relaxed hands than try to achieve more with tense, rigid hands.

3. Lifting and rotating the head

These movements will relax tension in the neck and throat. They increase rotation of the head and lengthen the upper spine.

Sit behind your partner's head and place both hands at the base of their skull. Slowly lift your partner's head up and their chin nearer their chest, thus extending the neck towards you and giving length to the upper spine.

From the same position slowly roll the head from side to side. You need to sense whether your partner is relaxed enough to let the head go freely.

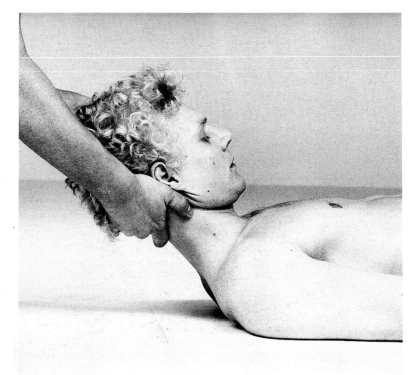

3

4. Stretching the neck

Put your left hand on your partner's left shoulder and your right hand under the base of the skull. Stretch the head towards you and push the shoulder away, rotating the head at the same time very gently.

Repeat the exercise with the right shoulder, rotating the head the opposite way.

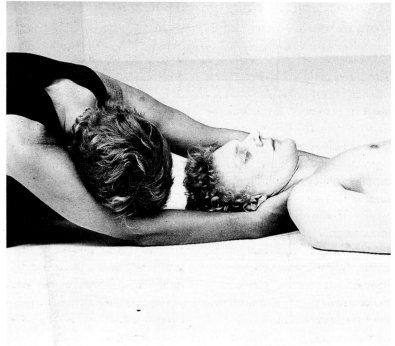

4

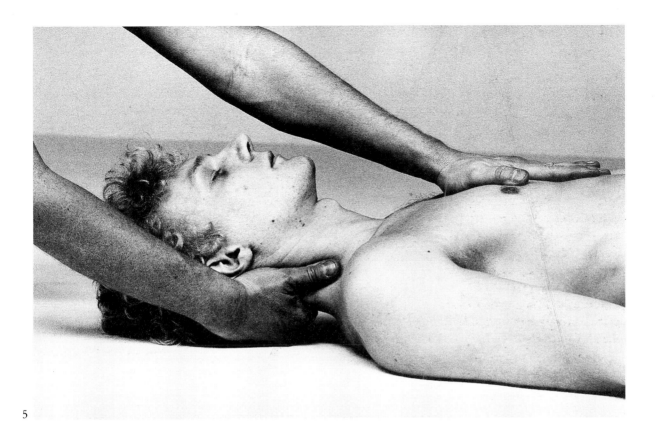

5

5. Connecting the energy from the head to the chest

This movement will increase your partner's breathing capacity. It also brings them in touch with the upper centre which is associated with consciousness, personal expression and the emotions. This often facilitates an emotional release. It is my favourite area of work – I feel I am touching the inner person.

Still sitting behind your partner's head, place your left hand on your partner's chest at the centre of the breastbone, with your fingers pointing downwards. Place the right hand under the base of the skull. The contact should be receptive and positive. Concentrate on feeling that your two bodies have become one, with energy flowing both ways. Again it is the idea of active non-doing. Pay attention to your partner's breathing and synchronize yours with theirs; be with the breath without actively doing anything. You should be able to feel the pulsing at the breastbone. Sense whether it is sluggish or over-active. Is the breath getting into the chest? Does the breath flow smoothly and slowly or is it dense and tightly held? Visualize the energy passing between your hands, opening a route for the expression of this energy.

Let your partner set the rhythm of the breathing pattern. When you fully feel a connection with your partner, gently push the chest down as you breathe out while at the same time lengthening the neck towards you. Do not push until they are well into the exhalation. You are trying to give them the experience of deeper, fuller breathing. After all the breath has been pushed out, pause an instant and then let your hand, still connected, ride up with the inhalation.

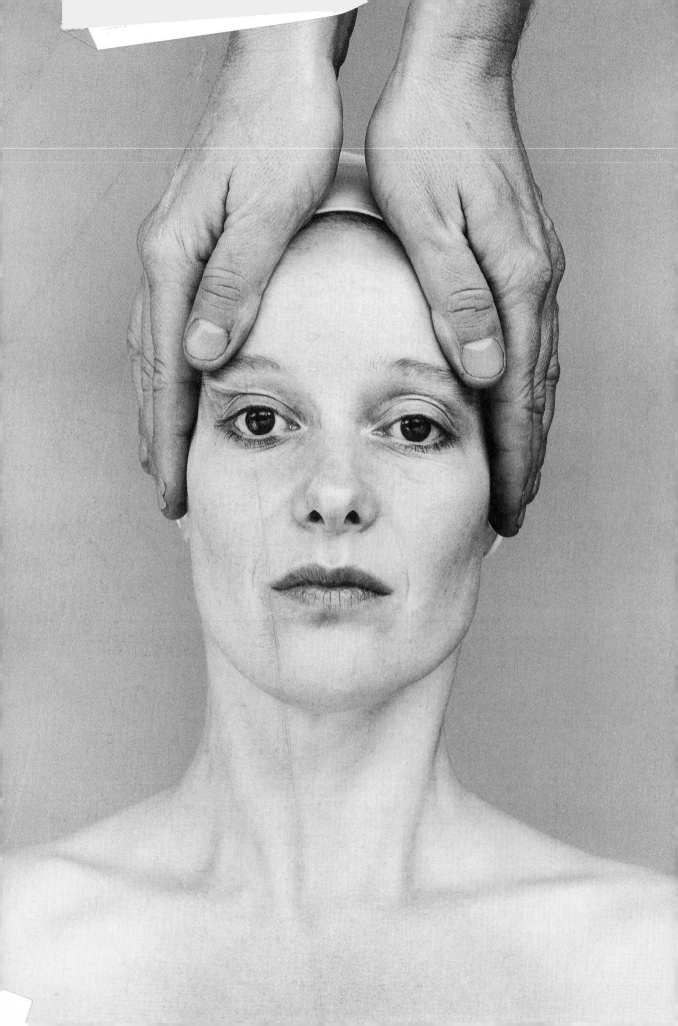

6. Facial massage strokes

The forehead and temples can get hot and lined with stress – in fact, the whole face can get very tense. These strokes should help to release the tension.

a) Sit at your partner's head – they can be sitting but it's better if they're lying down – and place both thumbs at the centre of the forehead. Your fingers should gently hold the head on either side. Use a soft strength to draw the thumbs outwards and down to the floor. Always take the strokes to their completion. Do this several times.

b) Stroke the cheekbones with both thumbs in a similar manner. Begin to learn about your own energy by sensing how softly or strongly you need to work. Massage with sensitivity and intuition; a positive presence is a gift.

c) Stroke the jawbone and chin with your thumbs. These are often held tight with unexpressed anger and emotion. This area is related to the pelvis and ankles, so if you find tension here you can expect to find it at the ankles as well.

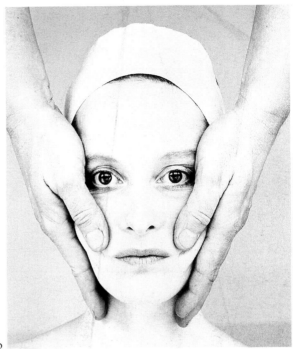

6b

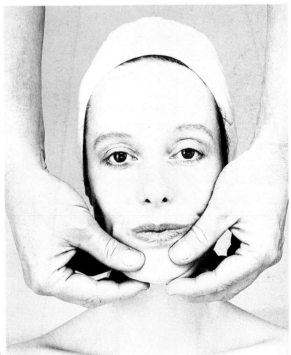

6c

6a

7. Stimulating the facial points

This technique is useful for stimulating perception generally and relieving headaches and nervous stress.

Using both thumbs, work the points at one-inch intervals from the centre of the forehead up over the top of the head. As the head is made up of over 20 bones fused together, it is quite soft and sensitive, so thumb pressure should be gentle, yet connected.

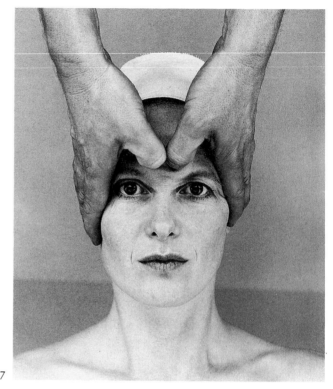

7

8. Warming the temples

In this movement you will be stimulating the gall bladder points. It will be especially helpful for relieving migraines.

With the heel of your hands on the temples, hold the sides of the face closely, imparting warmth. Visualize the energy passing between your hands. If you are able to picture what you are trying to effect, your treatment will be focused and felt with more depth.

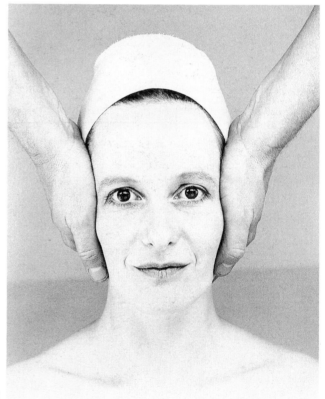

8

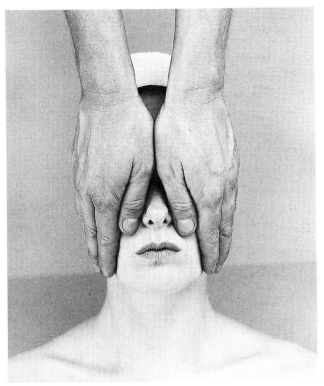

9

9. Covering the eyes

This calming technique takes your partner's energy down inside the body by shutting out any external visual stimulation and allowing you to transmit your energy into your partner. It also relaxes your partner's eye muscles and reduces nervous tension.

Cover your partner's eyes with your hands and simply hold the position with relaxed hands.

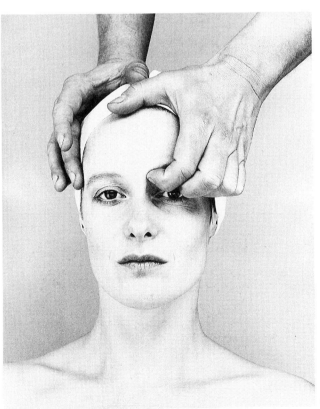

10

10. Working the eye points

This is done chiefly to reduce eye strain and can also relieve sinusitis.

You will be able to feel the edge of the bone that forms the eye socket – the bladder points are located here. Simply stimulate these points with your fingertips around the bone.

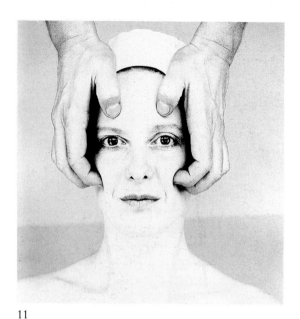

11

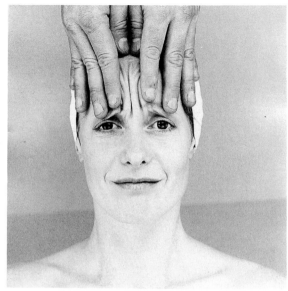

12

11. Working the nose and cheek points

This, together with the previous technique, helps to relieve sinusitis and it also improves the circulation of the blood in the face.

Using your fingertips, find the underside of the cheekbone at the side of the face. Press through the skin at various points along the edge of the bone moving towards the nose. Repeat this several times.

Then find the hollow beneath the cheekbone near the nose and, using your fingertips, press firmly with a relaxed hand. Repeat.

12. Stimulating the facial muscles

Massaging the muscles and stretching the loose tissue relaxes and improves the circulation of the blood in the face.

The face can be massaged in many different ways, so work at finding the best strokes for you, trusting your intuition to tell you what feels right. You can use opposition strokes, in which one hand works in the opposite direction to that of the other. If you do this, always finish with a long, smoothing stroke. Alternate strokes with your work on the points, as the strokes will have a calming effect after the focused intensity of the point work.

13. Lifting the skull

This exercise is the most effective quick relief from headaches and eye strain caused by tension and mental fatigue. It also aligns the spine, taking the strain off the superficial muscles of the neck that is caused by habitually tilting the head forwards. It should be done right at the end of the massage as it requires your partner to sit up. It is an invigorating, lifting technique and a good way to end the massage.

Sit, kneel or stand behind your partner who should be sitting in a relaxed position. If you are sitting you can support their spine with your knees, as in the shoulder stretch technique in the previous lesson (see p. 98). Place one hand on the forehead and the other, with the fingers slanting upwards, at the base of the skull. Lift the head straight up. The sense of lift comes from the lower hand whilst the hand on the forehead is for support and balance.

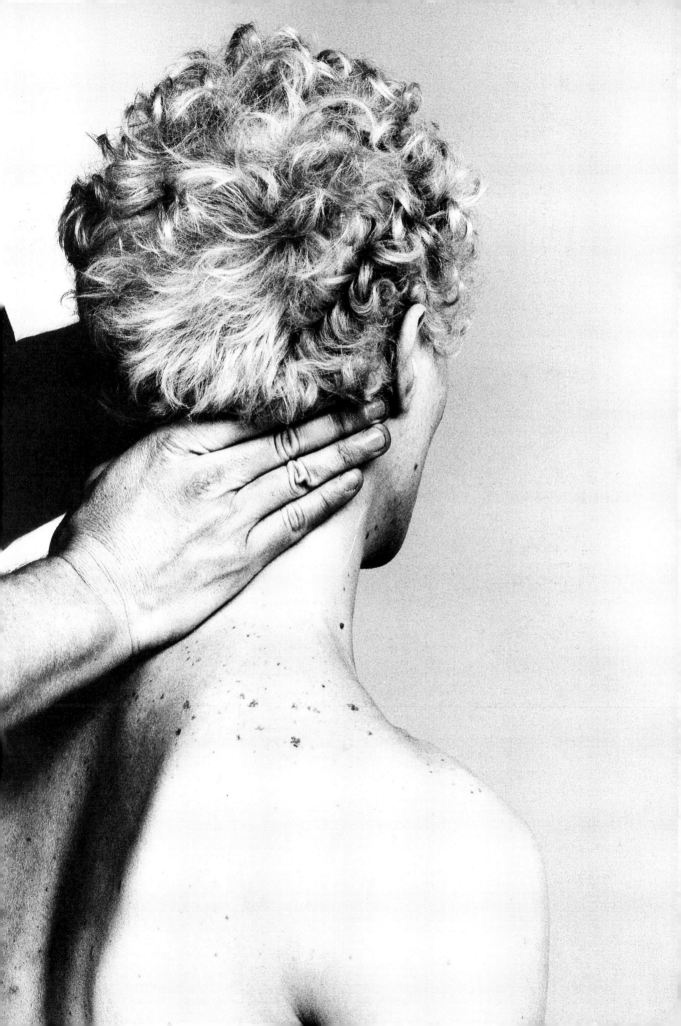

BODY READING

Our outward appearance is an expression of our inner life and maps a history of our relationship with the world. With the passing of time and the constant changes in our life, the way we look and move changes. Muscles are shaped by our patterns of movement, which respond to emotional and mental attitudes within. They become fixed and habitual – and easily recognizable by those around us. We are often too involved inside our own experiences to see our own patterns clearly. By observing others, however, we can learn about ourselves, increasing our range of understanding and our potential.

In massage, learning to be perceptive adds depth and dimension to our ability to assist others. It is important to watch – not to be always *doing*. We should develop patience, learn not to look too directly at a person but at the space around. Look for the obvious and for what is missing. We should not be too quick to define and judge what we think we see but should let clarity unfold, allowing time and space for change. The purpose of observing others is not to criticize. We must learn to look softly.

When we look at a person the first thing we see is the physical structure: shape, colour, texture and movement. Look at the body shape. Is it lengthened or dense? Does it seem well-proportioned? Is there a sense of openness at the chest? Is there excess energy in one area in relation to another? What is the relationship with the ground? Do the feet support the body? Is the weight centred and balanced? Are the feet turned out or directed forward? Are the thighs relaxed or tightly held and contained?

If the body's weight is thrown too far forwards onto the toes, so that the heel is not fully planted during walking, the image will be one of taking flight, as if the person fears the idea of their own physicality. Usually, such a body will be held together by tension, with an excess of energy. The person will move very quickly no matter what the task. But they need to feel their legs and sense the ground beneath their feet.

The opposite case is when the person pushes back into the heels. It is usually accompanied by a rolling in at the ankles, creating a look of insecurity and instability. The lack of upward energy often gives an air of defeat.

In a healthy and well-integrated body, the legs present a visual image of rootedness while the rest gives a sense of being lifted and energized upwards against the opposing pull of gravity. The upward lift and the body's sense of movement and direction need to be co-ordinated through a lengthened spine and head.

Watch the body movement. In what part of the body is movement initiated and how does it follow through? We are 90 per cent water and should move and change with a fluid quality. Is there vitality and a sense of purpose to the body movement? What does the face say? And what about the way the arms are held? Do they just hang lifelessly at the sides? What is the relationship between the right and the left side? Look at the body as a whole; the person may have a vibrant, strong quality, radiating energy, or be pale and weak with a low energy capacity.

We need to take the time to look and see what is actually there; to learn what the body tells us about the person within.

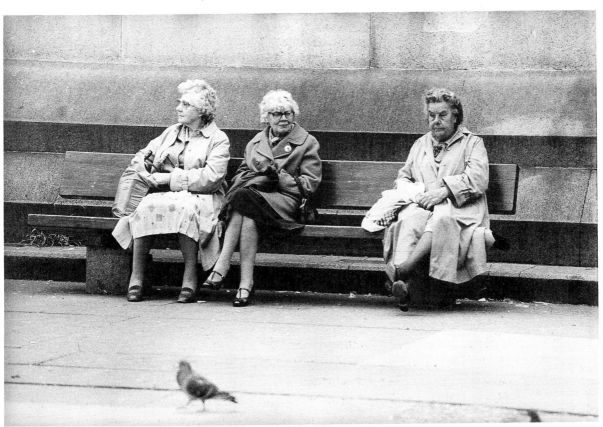

By observing others we can learn about ourselves

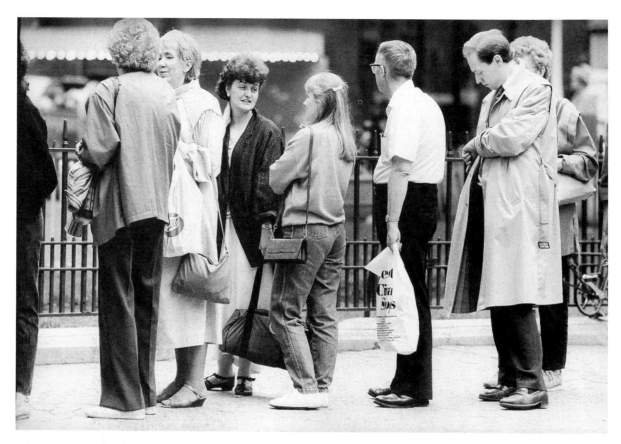

Above   In the photograph of a bus queue you can see body weight being carried in a variety of ways. Perhaps for the woman in jeans unevenly developed muscles make it more comfortable for her to stand on one leg and rest the other while, for the man with short sleeves, weak shoulder and back muscles make a heavy bag seem almost too much of a burden to carry.

Right   When a well-aligned body is viewed from the side, you should be able to draw a vertical line straight through the ear, shoulder joint, hip, knee and ankle.

The image here, however, is of the body being 'hung up' from behind the neck. The head falls towards the chest and the shoulders roll forward, the neck is compressed and the chest cavity collapses, cutting off the supply of breath. The pelvis also rolls forwards and the vital organs are displaced. (Hands in pockets give a good indication of this.) The knees are locked as the weight is pushed back onto the heels and the toes lift. Energy is held in the chest and shoulders, leaving the legs ungrounded. It is a look of instability, insecurity, even loss or defeat.

Following page, left   In a healthy, well-integrated body the head sits light and moves with freedom on the physical structure, allowing the face an expression of clarity, focus and vitality. The body, vertically lifted, moves with strength and purpose. Power is generated through the legs and expressed in the open chest and relaxed arms. The movement follows through in the co-ordination of the opposite arm and leg. She has not lost the spontaneity of childhood, yet has attained the depth and focus of maturity.

Following page, right   Without a positive relationship to gravity, life becomes an endless struggle. Excess energy appears to be contained in this man's chest, shoulders and throat, and his head is thrust forward. The body weight is thus top heavy, imposed on legs which offer little support. The lack of balance makes the movement unco-ordinated and the energy level is low. Dogged determination keeps him going.

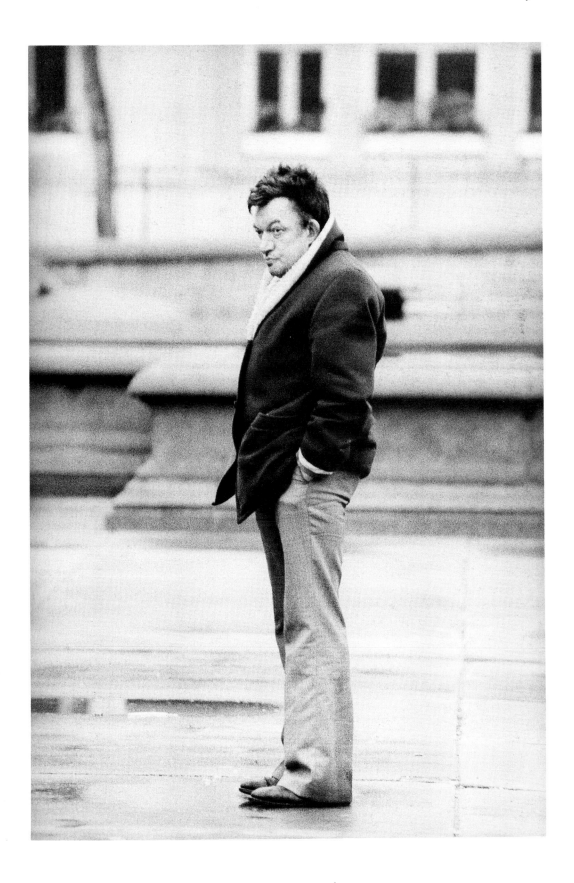

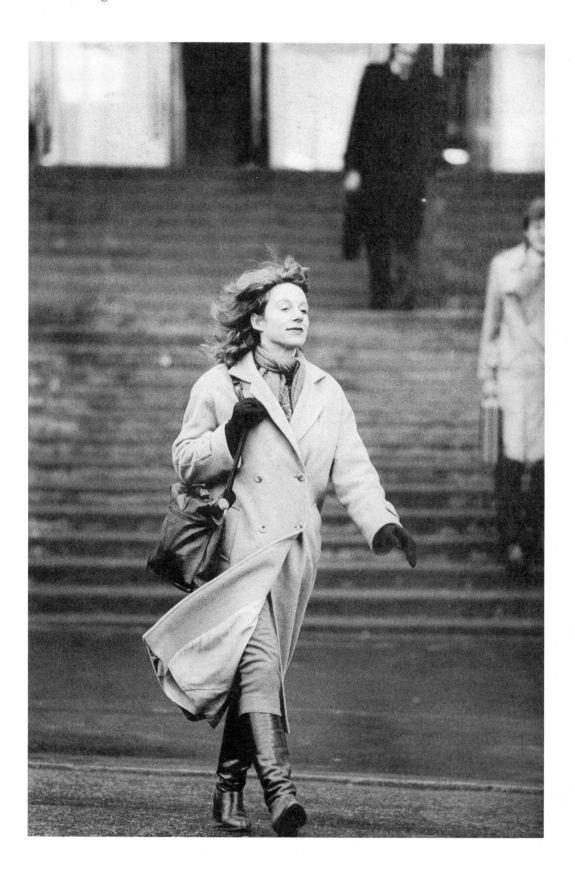

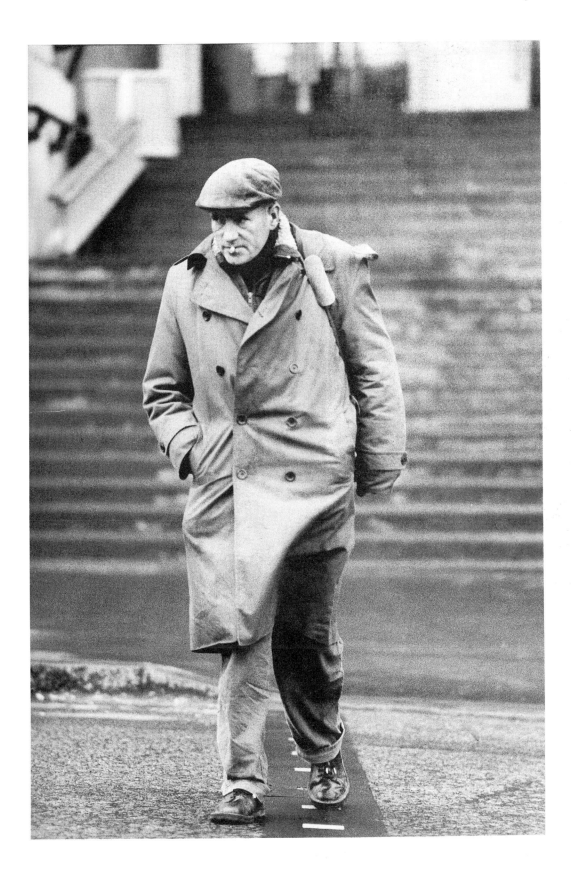

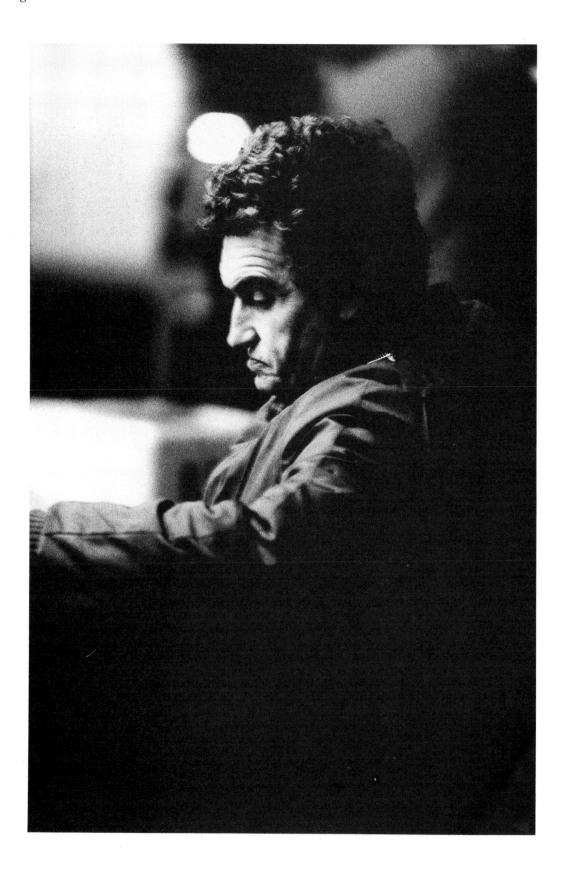

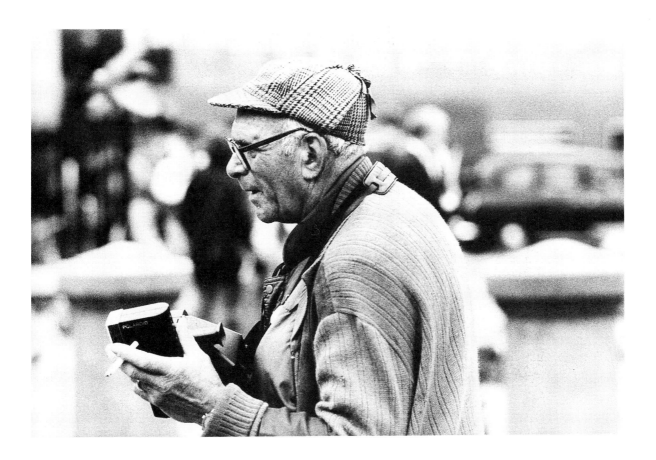

Left The face is a direct reflection of the heart. It gives an outward expression of our inner being, our general health, mental activity and emotions. It can be held in a fixed, angry look to keep others at a distance or show a build-up of deep emotion – sadness, loneliness, disappointment – without even knowing.

Above The photographer has a tense back with bound shoulders. Excess energy travels up the back, lifting and rounding them. From what we can see we know that the lower back and legs will be lacking in energy and ground connection. The bound shoulders leave the arms hanging weak and disconnected from a co-ordinated relationship with the rest of the body. The severe curve of the spine leaves the neck weak and vulnerable, limiting movement of the head and cutting off the supply of nutrition and oxygen to the brain. There will be a lack of physical and mental energy – even the camera around his neck seems too heavy for him to carry comfortably. Breathing will be shallow as the chest is collapsed.

Society has learnt to see all these signs of physical deterioration as the typical and inevitable characteristics of old age. They are, however, merely the visible result of a lifetime of bad posture and movement habits, making the natural process of ageing much worse than it need be.

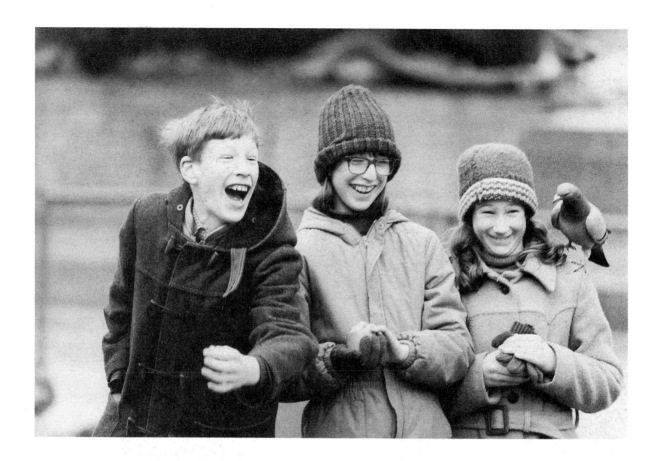

Above and right   Children radiate an alive and spontaneous presence that is relaxed, fluid and alert to change. They have a natural quality of ground and centre, generating energy upwards through a lengthened spine and well-positioned neck. They have not had time to develop bad movement habits and posture. It is interesting to note the group bonding in the group of three as the two girls lean against each other while holding their hands in a similar way.

The absence of tension in the upper body means children can react to the humour of a situation with a natural freedom and fluidity.

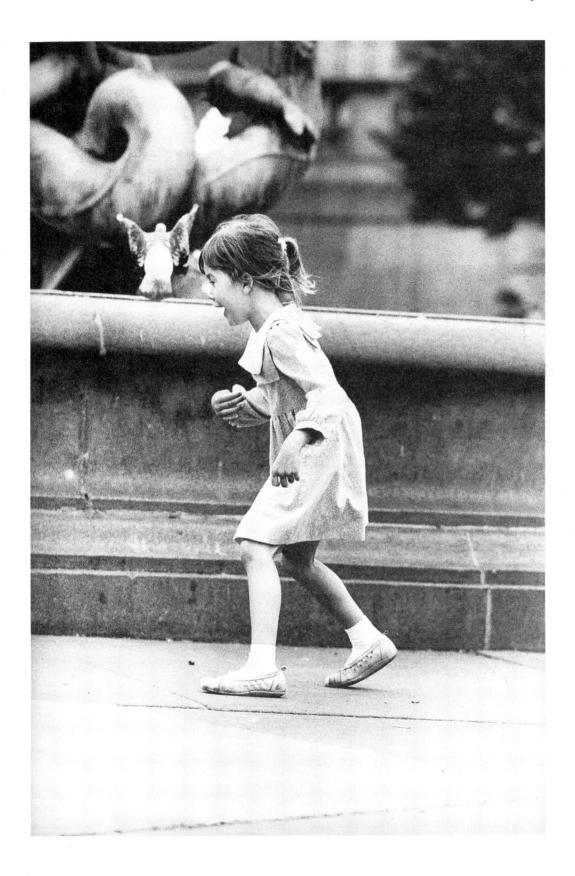

FURTHER READING

Capra, Fritjof, *The Tao of Physics*, Wildwood House, 1975

Chilton Pearce, Joseph, *Magical Child*, Paladin, 1979

Connelly, Dianne M., *Traditional Acupuncture: The Law of the Five Elements*, The Centre for Traditional Acupuncture, 1979

Elsworth Todd, Mabel, *Early Writings 1920–1934*, Dance Horizons, 1977

Feitus, Rosemary, *Ida Rolf Talks about Rolfing and Physical Reality*, The Rolf Institute, 1978

Feldenkrais, M., *Awareness Through Movement*, Harper and Row, 1972

Feldenkrais, M., *Body and Mature Behaviour: A Study of Anxiety, Sex, Gravitation and Learning*, International University Press, 1975

Kaptchuk, Ted J., *Chinese Medicine*, Rider, 1983

Keleman, Stanley, *Your Body Speaks its Mind*, The Center Press, 1981

Kurtz, Ron, and Prestera, Hector, MD, *The Body Reveals*, 1976

Lowen, Alexander, MD, *Bioenergetics*, Penguin Books, 1976

Masunaga, Shizuto and Wataru, Ohashi, *Zen Shiatsu*, Japan Publications, 1977

Payne, Peter, *Martial Arts: The Spiritual Dimension*, Thames and Hudson, 1981

Rolf, Ida P., *Rolfing: The Integration of the Human Structures*, Harper and Row, 1977

Strozze Heckler, Richard, *The Anatomy of Change*, Shambhala, 1984

Wataru, Ohashi, *Do-it-Yourself Shiatsu*, Unwin, 1976